Principles of Plant Pathology

NIPA® GENX ELECTRONIC RESOURCES & SOLUTIONS P. LTD.
New Delhi-110 034

About the Author

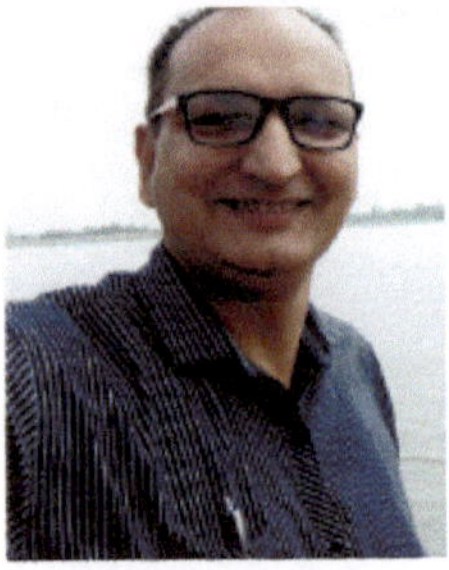

Dr. Sanjeev Kumar is an Assistant Professor in the Department of Plant Pathology, Jawaharlal Nehru Krishi Vishwavidyalaya, Jabalpur, Madhya Pradesh. He is a very sincere and enthusiastic teacher. He has taught with dedication to the satisfaction of students in many undergraduate, graduate and doctoral programs and has been actively involved in all educational activities. Dr. Kumar has mentored 20 MSc and 2 PhD students and is also actively involved in their research and extension activities. As a researcher, he has been involved in his eight major research projects sponsored by ICAR, NATP, TSP and JICA, Japan. He has published 75 research and review articles, 25 book chapters, 105 popular articles, 1 technical bulletin and 3 technical folders. He is an active member of more than six national and international societies. He is fellow of Indian Phytopathological Society, IARI New Delhi, Indian Society of Mycology and Plant Pathology, Udaipur, Rajasthan, Society for Biocontrol Advancement, Banglulu. He has participated in many conferences, symposiums, workshops and presented papers. He also attended the World Soybean Research Conference in Durban, South Africa. Dr. kumar has authored eight books entitled Plant Pathogens and Principles of Plant Pathology, Diseases of Horticultural Crop: Identification and Management, Diseases of Field Crop and Their Integrated Management, Pesticides and Plant Protection Appliances, Diseases of Field and Horticultural Crop Diseases and Their Management-II, Fundamentals of Plant Pathology, Integrated Disease Management; Principles & Practices published by New India Publishing Agency, Pithampura, New Delhi and Textbook of Diseases of Field and Horticultural Crop and Their Management-I published by, Brillion Publishing, Desh Bandhu Gupta Road, Karol Bagh, New Delhi-110005 and three practical manuals. His research interests include pulse pathology and biological control.

Principles of Plant Pathology
(As Per ICAR BSMA Syllabus)

Sanjeev Kumar
Assistant Professor
Department of Plant Pathology
Office of Dean, Faculty of Agriculture
Jawaharlal Nehru Krishi Vishwa Vidyalaya
Jabalpur-482004, Madhya Pradesh, India

NIPA® GENX ELECTRONIC RESOURCES & SOLUTIONS P. LTD.
New Delhi-110 034

NIPA, GENX ELECTRONIC
RESOURCES & SOLUTIONS P. LTD.

101,103, Vikas Surya Plaza, CU Block
L.S.C.Market, Pitam Pura, New Delhi-110 034
Ph : +91 11 27341616, 27341717, 27341718
E-mail:newindiapublishingagency@gmail.com
Website: www.nipabooks.com

For customer assistance, please contact
Phone: + 91-11-27 34 17 17
Fax: + 91-11-27 34 16 16
E-Mail: feedbacks@nipabooks.com

ISBN: 978-93-58870-82-4

Composed and Designed by NIPA®.

Preface

A paradigm shift in the higher agricultural education system has been found to be necessary in order to comply with the various provisions of the National Education Policy 2020. ICAR continues to work on the reforms needed to ensure the quality of agricultural education in India. The council appointed a national core group and BSMA committee to review and restructure the post graduate curriculum. The MSc(Ag)Plant Pathology syllabus has been revised and new courses have been introduced. The curriculum has been revised to enable students to acquire knowledge, approach entrepreneurship and improve their employability and skills to prepare for international competitiveness. This 'Principles of Plant Pathology' book has been carefully written for the PG class and is fully compliant with the latest syllabus. The purpose of writing this text book is to provide basic and fresh facts to enable students to introduce the scientific foundations of this course. Great care was taken to present facts appropriate to the student's level and grade the content accordingly. The text of the book is clear, well presented and arranged according to the curriculum. Infohive aims to inspire young minds to learn new things and expand their skills.Chapters are designed to lead to comprehensive learning, with key concepts to help students' to develop investigative skills.

I make no claims of originality in the creation of this book and have had the help of numerous books, magazines, bulletins, and electronic resources. We would like to express our sincere gratitude to the pioneers of past and present in the field of plant pathology.

The book entitled Principles of Plant Pathology written by me is dedicated to my parents, who sacrificed everything to give me the most and best education possible, to my wife, 'Archana' whose love and support have been the most precious things to me throughout our life together and who helped me in many facets of preparation of this and of previous books and finally, to "Saumya" and "Adyan" our youngest children who someday when they read their names in the book, may be reassured of "Papa" love for them and may feel proud of their father.

In this endeavor, omissions and errors will inevitably be found, and I accept responsibility for factual errors. Teachers and students are invited to comment on the book and make suggestions for further improvement.

Jabalpur, 2023

Sanjeev Kumar

Contents

Infohive

S.No.	Term	Description
1.	Aggressiveness	Descriptive of relative rate at which disease develop. Measure of reproductive fitness of pathogen while growing in/on the host.
2.	Deme system	Deme denotes a population of invidiuals within a specified taxon. Robinson (1969) observed that deme system should be reserved for host.
3.	Determinative control	System control which is imposed by man with aview to achieiving predetermined objectives. Deterministic control is a feature of all artificial (manmade) system ans is totally against all natural system.
4.	Differeential host	A series of vertical pathodemes used for the identification of vertical pathotypes. Ideally, each differential host should possess only one vertical gene.
5.	Differentail interation	When a series of different pathodeme is inoculated with a series of different pathotypes there is a differential interaction if more than one pathotype is necessary to differentiate the pathodeme and vice versa.
6.	Disease cycle	The cycle which starts with infection of the host and ends with reproduction of the pathogen.
7.	Disease escape	For normal disease development suitable combination of four elements of disease pyramid is required. If any one or more of these conditions do not coincide, disease may not develop.
8.	Disease square	The artificial , crop pathosystem in which there are four primary elements of systems control; the host ,the pathogen, and the environment and man.
9.	Disease triangle	A natural wild pathosystem in which there are only three primary elements of system control the host, the pathogen and the environment.
10.	Disease	The adverse effects on the host due to a pathogen (which lacks mouth parts) as opposed to damage which is due to a pest (which possesses a mouth parts)
11.	Dissemination efficiency	The ability of a parasite to disperse over wide areas in a short time.
12.	Duster	This is an equipment used for the distribution of finely powdered material.
13.	Epidemic cycle	The positive growth of a parasite population from minimum to maximum followed by a negative growth to minimum. Most epidemic cycle are seasonal.

14.	Epidemiological competence	The ability of a parasite to survive and hence to cause an epidemic in a particular environment.
15.	Esodemic	That part of the epidemic which is due to autoinfection.
16.	Exodemic	That parts of the epidemic which is due to alloinfection.
17.	Facultative parasite	A parasite which is also able to grow saprophytically.
18.	Homeostasis	The ability of a dynamic system both to maintain a stable optimum and to return to that optimum in the events of a loss of system balance.
19.	Immunity	An immune plant is non host. Immunity is an absolute quality. It is a variable survival value.A plant is either immune or it is not immune to a parasite. Anything less than immunity is resistance which is a variable survival value.
20.	Isozymes	Different proteins with distinct genetic origins that catalyze the same reaction. It catalyze the same reaction. Their effect may vary quantitatively that is one isozyme may be more efficient catalytically than another. The product however stays the same that is there is no qualitative difference in product.
21.	Macroevolution	It involves population changes due to selection pressure. These changes involves characters which are new. They are not reversibleand they normally occur over a period of geological time.
22.	Markov chain	A multidecision process in which every decision is entirely random and is independent of any previous decision.
23.	Microevolution	Involves changes which are not new which are reversible and which occurs over periods of historical time (in month, in year)
24.	Multiline	A multiline is a mixture of phenotypically similar but genotypically dissimilar pure lines. The genotypic differences usually involve vertical resistance. A multiline is a plant pattern of vertical resistance.
25.	Multiple resistance	The resistance is one organisms of a no of various major genes and or polygenes which independently result in resistance to different group of pesticides.
26.	Natural pathosystem	A pathosystem in a natural, wild ecosystem in which there has been no interference of man.
27.	Negative cross resistance	A mutation in one gene leads to resistance to one pesticide and increased sensitivity to other.
28.	Negative positive rule	The rule that , in screening a flexible host population.
29.	Negative screening	Negative screening is a type of screening done before flowering.
30.	Obligate parasite	A parasite which is unable to grow saprophytically.
31.	Oligogenic resistance	Resistance whose inheritance is controlled by few genes. Vertical resistance is always oligogenic resistance but not all oligogenic resistance is vertical.

32	Parasite	An organism which depends on a living host for it nutrient but which does not normally destroy that host in the way that a predator destroy its prey. Parasites are usually classified either as; Pathogen: which lacks mouth parts or Pest : which possess mouth parts.
33.	Parasitic ability	The ability of a parasite to survive at the expense of its host.
34.	Parasitism	Phenomenon of a parasite surviving at the expense of its host. The definitive characteristic of a pathosystem.
35.	Pathodeme	A population of host species in which all individuals have a stated pathosystem character (resistance) in common. Hence vertical pathodeme , horizontal pathodeme etc.
36.	Pathogen	A parasite which has no mouth parts and which is studied by a plant pathologists (fungi, bacteria, virus) used in opposition to pest which is usually defined as a parasitic eating the host by means of mouth parts.
37.	Pathogenicity	Ability of a pathogen to survive at the expense of its host.
38.	Pathosystem management	The determinative control of crop pathosystem in order to reduce crop loss due to parasites to a minimum without reducing yield, or quality , without affecting crop uniformity in space and time without cost ot the farmer and without crop vulnerability.
38.	Pathosystem manager	A multidisciplinary plant scientist who is primarily interested in effective pathosystem management.
39.	Pathosystem	Any subsystem of an ecosystem which involes parasitism. A pathosystem may be Natural- wild pathosystem-Disease triangle Artificial- Crop pathosystem- Disease square
40.	Pathotype	A population of parasite species in which all individuals have a stated pathosystem character (pathogenicity or parasitic ability) in common. Hence vertical pathotype, Horizontal pathotypes)
41.	Pest	A plant parasite with mouth parts.
42.	Physiologic specialization	Any differential interaction between pathodems and pathotypes.
43.	Plant esodemic	The esodemic at the pathosystem level of one host individual. The plant esodemic involves autoinfection within the component of that one individual.
44.	Plant exodemic	The exodemic at the pathosystem level of host individual . The plant exodemic involves allo infection between individuals.
45.	Polyphyletic resistance	Any apparent immunity which however can be genetically diluted by hybridization of the host.
46.	Polyphyletic	Means multiple origin. A polyphyletic host or parasite is derived by hybridization.
47.	Positive cross resistance	A mutation in one gene leads not only to resistance against pesticide under consideration but also to pesticides to which the same resistance mechanism applies.
48.	Positive screening	Positive screening is the type of screening done before, during, and/or after harvesting.

49.	Qualitative resistance	Horizontal resistance is qualitative in its inheritance, its mechanism and its effect when it is inherited oligogenic ally. V.R is qualitative when its confer complete protection against non-matching vertical pathotypes. A polyphylectic pathosystem may also be qualitative.
50.	Resistance	Genetic ability to prevent, check or slow down (resist) the activities of a known pathogen of the plant species.
51.	Screening	A means of exerting selection pressure on a genetically flexible population.Screening may be Positive: retention of desirable individual. Negative: rejection of undesirable character.
52.	Sprayer	This is a machine in which the liquid is broken up into fine droplets and ejected under pressure. The aim of spraying is to apply a pattern of discreate droplets.
53.	Surveillance	Synonymous with monitoring meaning close and usually continuous observation of a subject in this instance a crop for the detection of the presence of pathogens and determination of their population density, dispersion and dynamics.
54.	Survey	A survey is a planned activity which measures and records factors observed, either over a single period or over a extended period of time.
55.	Susceptible	Lack of resistance.
56.	Tolerance	Genetic ability to tolerate pathogen and its activities without showing significant yield losses, at a given level of disease severity.

1

Plant Pathology: Definition, Objectives, Scope and Importance

Prologue: The Issues

Farmers lose a significant portion of their income when their crops and products become infested with various insects, diseases and weeds, resulting in much lower crop productivity and lower actual yields than the attainable yield of crops. Yield losses due to pests, pathogens and weeds are responsible for 20-40% losses in global agricultural productivity. India reports crop losses of 20-25% annually due to pest infestations. Without the use of crop protection solutions, there could be a 78% loss in fruit production, 54% loss in vegetable production and 32% loss in cereal production. According to the Ministry of Agriculture, India loses INR 1.48 billion worth of agricultural production annually due to pests, weeds and plant diseases.

Climate change is an important development that has affected global population and agriculture. Complexity of diseases is likely to increase, with more frequent disease outbreaks. Disease dynamics have altered considerably. Many minor diseases have become major diseases and many new diseases have emerged. This has kept the plant pathology sector on their toes.

Although a wide range of crop protection measures exist, chemicals are synonymous with plant disease management. Although the effectiveness of crop protection products are undisputed, their continued and indiscriminate use far outweighs their benefits, and their side effects have received a lot of attention. There have been strengths and opportunities for updating existing approaches of disease management. The result was adoption of integrated disease management and chemical means of disease management became one of its many components.

Of late, much of modern research in plant pathology aims at finding other environmentally friendly means of controlling plant diseases. The most promising approaches include conventional breeding and genetic engineering of disease-resistant plants, application of disease-suppressing cultural practices,

RNAand gene-silencing techniques of plant defense promoting nontoxic substances and to some extent, use of biological agents antagonistic to the microorganisms that cause plant disease. Resistance is the first line of defense against invading pathogens. In addition to conventional breeding, genetic engineering has also achieved excellent results. Plant disease prediction is an underutilized area in India. Pests and diseases are highly dependent on weather variables, and many models have been developed to predict disease outbreaks. However, in conventional agriculture these models are rarely used. However, in the next few years, model-based forecasting will gain momentum in plant pathology. Biopesticides and biocontrol agents represent another aspect of crop protection. This is becoming all the more important given the determination of many Indian states to go fully organic. Nanotechnology is a fascinating and rapidly evolving science that is used in plant protection has the potential to revolutionize many areas of.

We have around 14 crores of farmers in more than six lakhs villages in India. Reaching out to them by any individual or institutions is impossible. This gloomy picture has been fortunately changing since 2015 due to modern technology. Digital tools are one of the most innovative crop protection tools of modern agriculture. Technologies like mobile application, artificial intelligence (AI), internet of things (IoT), big data, robot, and predictive analysis among others have streamlined the supply chain system. This has ensured holistic risk management of farmers and helped them to get the right price for their produce. In present scenario, with the use of smart phones, one can take the technology to a large number of farmers inhabited in remote areas. Through the availability of smart phones, farmers can find the right solutions to their problems by downloading certain apps, or they can reach easily to companies and scientists like us by sending images regarding their problems to get the accurate solutions. So, in this way, digitization can help farmers to a large extent. We are still at a nascent stage but internationally, all the data comes through satellites and they are very much precise in agriculture. Overall, digitisation could help farmers in getting technology at their doorsteps eg- weather forecasting, prediction of diseases in advance, projection of insect attack, estimation of market prices etc. would be very helpful to the farmers. Teachers and students need to be trained about digital tools. To address these changes in teaching methodologies, University need support to introduce teaching excellence tools for faculty and students.

Crop protection measures are only available towards the end of each package of practices they ultimately determine crop health and quantity. Investing in proper crop protection measures is therefore a very smart and sensible way to sustainable agriculture . Public and private sectors will be keen on investing in better delivery techniques and products that leave very little impact on the plant and the soil.

Plant Pathology

The term plant pathology is derived from greek words- *pathos* (suffering) + *Logos* (study) i.e. the study of the suffering plant. Plant Pathology has two phases broadly-

- **Science-** *understanding of the disease* i.e. the theoretical consideration of the suffering plants and *how do pathogens invade, how do plants defend themselves, what causes symptoms etc.*
- **Art-** *the application of the science to the field problems* i.e. diagnosis and control.

Plant pathology or phytopathology is the branch of agricultural, botanical or biological science which deals with the cause, etiology, resulting in losses and management methods of plant diseases.

Plant pathology is a science that studies plant diseases and attempts to improve the chances for survival of plants when they are faced with unfavorable environmental conditions and parasitic microorganisms that cause disease. Plant pathology is so challenging, fascinating, important, and worth studying on its own. However, it is also a science that works to safeguard the food that is accessible to both people and animals.

Plant pathology is an integrative science and profession that uses and combines fundamental knowledge of botany, mycology, bacteriology, virology, nematology, plant anatomy, plant physiology, genetics and molecular biology and genetic engineering, biochemistry, horticulture, agriculture, tissue culture, soil science, forestry, chemistry, physics, meteorology, and many other scientific fields. Plant pathology has benefited from advances in each of these sciences, and many advances have been made in other sciences to solve plant pathological problems.

As a science, plant pathology seeks to improve our knowledge of plant diseases. At the same time, plant pathology seeks to develop methods, devices, and materials that can be used to prevent plant diseases or controlled. Uncontrolled crop diseases can lead to food shortages, higher food prices, or lower food quality. Affected plant products may be toxic and unsuitable for consumption. Some plant diseases may wipe out entire plant species, many of which affect beauty and landscape of our environment. Although plant disease control results in better quality food and a more aesthetically pleasing environment, consumers must pay for the cost of materials, equipment, and labor used to control plant diseases, and sometimes other less obvious costs of such as contamination of the environment.

Major objectives

- To study biotic, mesobiotic and abiotic causes of diseases or disorders.
- To study the mechanisms of disease development by pathogens.
- To study the plant (host)-pathogen interaction in relation to environment.
- To develop methods of management of plant diseases.

Scope of plant pathology

- Field surveys to determine disease prevalence and incidence.
- Recordings of newly emerging diseases of economic importance, including details and extent of outbreaks.
- Assessment of losses due to various economically important diseases.
- Studies of the etiology, symptoms, predisposition, and recurrence of such diseases.
- Identification of suitable and economical methods to managme economically important crop diseases.
- Support for breeding disease-resistant varieties.
- Training of advisors and subject matter experts to bridge the gap between pathologists and farmers for better crop production.

Importance of plant pathology in agriculture

- Plant pathology has advanced the knowledge to protect the crop from losses due to diseases.
- Most of the diseases with known disease cycle can now be avoided by the modification of cultural practices.
- With the knowledge of mode of disease spread, many diseases of economic importance can now be managed .
- Crop improvement and varietal resistance have been achieved against many diseases through the joint effort of breeder and plant pathologist.
- The science of plant pathology has contributed disease free certified seed production.

- Plant pathology has made it possible to limit the spread of plant diseases from one place to another and from one country to another through appropriate measures and quarantine laws.
- Knowledge of plant pathology allows various preventive measures to be taken to successfully treat disease. These measures are seed treatments, soil treatments and crop rotation.
- Diseases in cold storage can be avoided by taking phytopathological measures, following various disease management recommendations to protect stored fruits and vegetables.
- Plant pathology has enabled bioagents to be recognized, and utilized through toxicant production, competition and parasitism. Organisms that exert such lethal or harmful effects on other organisms are called antagonists.

Challenges for plant pathology

The challenges for plant pathology are

- To reduce food losses.
- To improve food quality.
- To safeguarde our environment.

2

Plant Diseases
Definitions, Importance and Concepts

Disease is one of those terms that are very difficult to define. It is realized that disease (literally *dis-ease*) implies *lack of 'comfort'* and therefore, involves *deviation from normal functioning*. From time to time several definitions which have been proposed, in fact descriptive but not simultaneously exclusive. The definitions for the term disease are:

- *Disease is a malfunctioning process that is caused by continuous irritation, which results in some suffering producing symptoms.*
- *Disease is an alteration in one or more of the ordered sequential series of physiological processes culminating in a loss of coordination of energy utilization in a plant as a result of the continuous irritation from the presence or absence of some factor or agent.*
- *Disease is any morphological or physiological abnormality in a plant or any of its parts caused by continuous irritation and results in economic losses to human beings.*
- *Any deviation from normal growth or structure of plants that is sufficiently pronounced and permanent to produce visible symptoms or to impair quality and economic value.*
- *A plant is said to be diseased when there is a harmful deviation from normal functioning of physiological process .*

All these definitions indicate that disease;

- Is not a pathogen but it is *caused by a pathogen.*
- It is not symptom but *results in symptoms.*
- It is not a condition as the condition results from disease and is not synonymous with it.
- It is *not an injury.*
- Cannot be infectious, it is actually the pathogen which is infectious.

- Results from continuous irritation.
- Disease is a malfunctioning process and this result in some suffering and therefore disease is a *pathological process*

Disease *Vs* Injury

- Disease occurs whenever a vital process in the host plant is continuously disrupted.
- Disease is particularly severe when the regulated intake and use of energy is impaired.
- Injury is sometimes confused with disease, and injurious agents are sometimes confused with pathogens. However, this confusion can be avoided.
- Injuries occur when plants are temporarily disturbed. E.g.. By mowers or grasshoppers.
- In contrast, disease occurs when plants are exposed to long-term injury or damage (or, as some authors prefer, "continuous irritation") by pathogens. Examples include wilt fungus and yellow spot fungus.

Concept of disease in plants

It is difficult to pinpoint exactly when a plant is diseased because it is not known whether plants feel pain or discomfort and because, in any case, plants do not speak or otherwise communicate with us.

Healthy Plant

- A plant is healthy, or normal, when it can carry out its physiological functions to the best of its genetic potential.
- The meristematic cells of a healthy plant divide and differentiate as required, and different types of specialized cells absorb water and nutrients from the soil; translocate these to all plant parts; carry on photosynthesis, translocate, metabolize, or store the photosynthetic products; and produce seed or other reproductive organs for survival and multiplication.

Diseased Plant

- When the ability of the cells of a plant or plant part to carry out one or more of these essential functions is interfered with by either a biotic or abiotic agents, the activities of the cells are disrupted, altered, or inhibited, the cells malfunction or die, and the plant becomes diseased.

- At first, the infection is localized to one or a few cells and is invisible. Soon, the reaction becomes more widespread and affected plant parts develop changes visible to the naked eye. These visible changes are symptoms of the disease.
- Visible or measurable detrimental changes in plants in response to biological infection or adverse environmental factors are measures of the degree of plant disease.
- Plant diseases can therefore be defined as a series of invisible responses of plant cells and tissues to biotic or abiotic agents. This can adversely affect plant morphology, function, or integrity, leading to partial plant failure or death.
- The type of cells and tissues affected determines the type of physiology that is disrupted first.
- Infection of roots might cause roots to rot and cause them to not able to soak up water and nutrients from the soil.
- Infection of xylem vessels, as takes place in vascular wilts and in a few cankers, interferes with the translocation of water and minerals to the crown of the plant.
- Infection of the foliage, as takes place in leaf spots, blights, rusts, mildews, mosaics, and so on, interferes with photosynthesis.
- Infection of phloem cells inside the veins of leaves and within side the bark of stems and shoots, as takes place in cankers and in diseases because of viruses, mollicutes, and protozoa, interferes with the downward translocation of photosynthetic products.
- Infection of flowers and fruits result interferes with reproduction.
- Although infected cells in most diseases are weakened or die, in a few diseases, e.g., infected cells are prompted to divide much faster (hyperplasia) or to make bigger a excellent deal extraordinary amorphous overgrowths (tumors) or abnormal organs.
- Pathogenic microorganisms which can cause disease/ailment are commonly called pathogens, commonly cause ailment in plants via way of means of disturbing the metabolism of plant cells via enzymes, toxins, growth regulators, and different materials they secrete and via way of means of absorbing foodstuffs from the host cells for his or her personal use.

- Some pathogens may additionally reason diseases via way of means of developing and multiplying within the xylem or phloem vessels of plants, thereby blockading the upward transportation of water or the downward motion of sugars, respectively, via those tissues.
- Environmental elements reason disease in plants whilst abiotic elements, which include temperature, moisture, mineral, nutrients, and pollutants, arise at stages above or beneath a certain range tolerated by plants

Importance of plant diseases

- Crop diseases can occur throughout the crop production chain and remain one of the greatest threats to the sustainable development of society. The result is a 13% to 22% reduction in annual yield or costing billions of dollars in economic costs in staple of rice wheat, corn and potatoes plus additional costs for research and development of management strategies.
- Plant diseases caused by infectious pathogens have had a profound impact on human society and nature throughout human history through damage to food production, economic development, ecosystem resilience and natural landscapes.
- Famine and malnutrition in Ireland caused by *Phytophthora infestans* (Mont.) de Bary, the pathogen of potato blight, and *Bipolaris oryzae* (Breda de Haan), the pathogen of rice brown spot famine in Bengal, led to millions of deaths and uprooted families and social structures.
- The pandemic of chestnut wilt pandemic caused by *Cryphonectria parasitica* (Murrill) Barr and dutch elm caused by *Ophiostoma novo-ulmi* (Buism.) Nann. destroyed much of the primary and secondary forestry industry in North America and Europe, causing an ecological disaster in the region.
- Plant diseases make plants toxic to humans and animals. Many plant pathogens produce mycotoxins that directly or indirectly threaten human and animal health.
- These biological and economic losses are responsible, at least in part, for the latest estimates of about 800 million people worldwide suffering from hunger or malnutrition.
- Plant diseases can also limit the variety of local crops and industries and reduce the quality and quantity of plant products.
- The costs of controlling crop diseases are also direct disease losses.

3

History and Growth of Plant Pathology

History of plant pathology records chronological account of important events, contributions of persons who significantly influenced the thinking of their era and interpretation of the observed facts or phenomenon over a period of time. Historical writings help us to understand systematic development in plant pathology, and there problems faced by certain outstanding workers whose view points were unacceptable to majority of opinion makers, simply because it was new and against the established norms of the day. History of plant pathology is a must read for the students of this discipline. The historical accounts will unfold the stories that may motivate the new generation to think and interpret the findings in their own way, without fear of established theories and dogmas carried from the past.

Development of Mycology

Year	Contributor (s)	Description
Around 750 BC	Theophrastus	• Plant diseases as the wrath of gods.
1500	Surapal	• Wrote 'Vraksha Ayurveda', the first book in which plant diseases were discussed.
1623	Gaspard Bauhin	• Written Pinax Theatri Botanici.
1665	Robert Hook	• Observed cell first time in microscope. • First observed Teliospore of *Pharagmidium disciflorum* under microscope.
1675	Anton von Leeuwenhoek	• Invented compound microscope.
1707-1778	C Linnaeus	• Written a book entitled Species Plantarum.
1729	PA Michaeli	• Studied fungi and saw their spores on the pieces of water melon. • Wrote '*Nova Plantarum Genera.* • Known as Father of Mycology.
1743	John Needham	• Reported plant parasitic nematodes in wheat galls.
1755	M Tillet	• Demonstrated that the bunt of wheat was contagious thought that the spores contained a poisonous entity. • Dusting of black smut powder in wheat seeds resulted in smutted heads.

Year	Contributor (s)	Description
1793	CH Persoon	• Produced '*Synopsis Methodica Fungorum'* • Considered as major starting point for nomenclature of rusts, smuts and Gausteromycetes.
1807	B Prevost	• Studied wheat bunt disease for about decade. • Published his result of studies as *Memoir on the intermediate cause of bunt or smut of wheat and of several diseases of plants, and on preventives of bunt.* • Confirmed findings of Tillet. • Proofed the role of a micro organism in the causation of disease. • Demonstrated the control of wheat smut by steeping seed in copper sulphate solution • Distinguished between fungicidal and fungistatic effects. • Prevost's results and interpretations were not accepted due to hold of the theory of spontaneous generatiaon at that time. • It has to wait some 40 years , only after the adoption of germ theory that Prevost's work was recognized.
1821	EM Fries	• Reported that smut and rust fungi as product of diseased plants. • Wrote " Systema Mycologium." • Known as Linnaeus of Mycology.
1827	Cragie	• Showed function of Puccinia in rust fungi.
1840	LR Tulasne & C Tulasne	• Confirmed the observation of Prevost with regard to the causal organism of wheat bunt. • Known as Reconstructor of Mycology
1858	JG Kuhn	• Published first text book on Plant Pathology namely "The Diseases of Cultivated Crops: Their causes and Their Control."
1860	Louis Pasteur	• Furnished evidence that *microroganisms arise from pre existing microorganisms.* • His discovery of bacterial origin of anthrax buried the theory of spontaneous generation forever.
1861-65	Anton de Bary	• First to indicate the nature of obligate and facultative forms. • Proved the real cause of late blight of potato is *Phytophthroa infestans*. • Described the sex and account of development in number of Phycomycetes and Ascomycetes. • Described the role of enzymes in plant diseases. • Demontrated heterocious nature of stem rust of wheat. • Wrote his famous text *Morphologie und Physiologie der pilze , Flechten , Und Myxomyceten.* • Known as the father of plant pathology.
1875	O Brefeld	• Developed pure culture technique.
1878	MS Woronin	• Discovered the life cycle of potato wart disease

Year	Contributor (s)	Description
1881	HM Ward	• Reported the role of environment in the epidemiology of coffee rust. • He is known as Father of Tropical Plant Pathology.
1882	Robert Hartig	• Published a textbook -Diseases of Trees. • He is called as "Father of Forest Pathology".
1885	PM Millardet	• Discovered the Bordeaux mixture for the control of downey mildew of grapes.
1885	Frank	• Discovered Mycorrhizal fungi.
1887	Mason	• Introduced Burgundy mixture.
1887	Jensen	• Developed hot water technique for management of wheat smut.
1894	Ericsson	• Reported physiological specialization in stem rust of wheat.
1904	AF Blakeslee	• Founded heterothallism in *Rhizopus*.
1905	RH Biffen	• First to show that resistance to pathogens in plants can be inherited as a Mendelian character.
1917	EC Stakman	• Distinguished biological forms in cereal rusts.
1923	Hansen and Smith	• Term Heterokaryosis.
1931	PA Saccardo	• Wrote "Syllogue Fungorum"
1931	JC Luthra	• Solar heat treatment for loose smut of wheat.
1940	KO Mullar and H Borger	• Studied hypersensitive response in potato phytophthora system and formally proposed the phytoalexin hypothesis.
1946	HH Flor	• Gave gene for gene hypothesis while working on linseed rust.
1950	AHR Buller	• Described sexual process in uredinales. Studied physiology of fungi and mechanism of spore discharge in fungi.
1951	Hotson and Cutter	• Artificial culturing of apple cedar rust (*Gymnosporangium juniperi-virginianae*).
1952	G Pontecorvo and JA Roper	• Discovered parasexuality in *Aspergillus nidulans*
1953	EC Large	• Introduced the term pathometry or phyto-pathometry for disease assessment and or disease measurement.
1968	Vander Plank	• Concept of horizontal and vertical resistance. • He is known as Father of Plant Epidemiology.
1990	DF Klessig and I Raskin; JP Metraux and J Tyals	• Demonstrated that salicylic acid is associated with systemic acquired resistance.
2005	RA Dean and Co-workers	• The first complete genome sequencing of a plant pathogenic fungus *Magnaporthe grisea*

Development of Plant Bacteriology

Year	Contributor (s)	Description
1683	Anton von Leeuwenhoek	• First observed bacteria.
1876	Robert Koch	• Established germ theory in relation to diseases of man and animals. • Proved that anthrax disease of cattle was caused by • specific bacterium. • Established Koch's postulates
1876	Louis Pasteur	• Demonstrated role of bacteria in fermentation and decay.
1876	Woronin.	• Isolated and described the root nodule bacteria in leguminous plant.
1879	Prilleaux	• Reported the bacterial decay of wheat kernels.
1880	TJ Burrill	• Proved that Fire blight of pear was caused by bacterium which he named *Micrococcus amylovorus*.
1883	JH Wakker	• Investigated yellow slime disease of hyacinth caused by bacterium.
1885-1887	JC Arther	• Confirmed Burrill's work.
1887	EF Smith	• Gave the final proof that bacteria could be the incitants of plant diseases. • First to notice and study the crown gall disease. • Father of Phytobacteriology.
1980	DW Dye and Co-workers	• Introduced pathovar system in taxonomy.
1910	CO Jensen	• Related crown gall of plants to cancer of animals.
1952	J Lederberg	• Coined the term plasmid.
1952	SA Waksman	• Discovered streptomycin.
1952	N D Zinder & J Lederberg	• Discovered transduction in bacteria.
1962	H Stolp	• Discovered bdellovibrios.
1972	PB New and A Kerr	• Success in biological control of *A. radiobacter* strain K.
1972	IM Windsor and LM Black	• Observed a new kind of phloem inhabiting bacterium causing clover club leaf disease.
1974	I. Zanen Co-workers	• Demonstrated Ti plasmid in *Agrobacterium tumefaciens*.
1977	Chilton and Co-workers	• Showed that the crown gall bacterium transforms normal plant cells into tumor cells by introducing into them a plasmid, part of which becomes inserted into the plant cell chromosomes DNA.
1980	DW Dye Co-workers	• Introduce pathovar system in taxonomy.

Development of Phytonematology

Year	Contributor (s)	Description
1743 AD	Needham	• First reported association of nematode with plant disease. • Described the wheat gall nematode caused by *Anguina tritici.*
1857	C Devaine	• Studied life cycle of *Anguina tritici.*
1855	MJ Berkley	• Noticed gall/knots on roots of cucumber. • Observed white larvae and eggs of the nematode and called them vibrio.
1875	Cornu	• First specific mention of root knot nematode. • Described under the name *Anguillula marioni.*
1887	EA Goeldi	• Published a description of *Meloidogyne exigua* (Coffee root knot).
1889	Atkinson	• Published preliminary report on lifecycle of nematode under the name *Heterodera radicicola.*
1857	Kuhn	• Reported stem nematode (*Ditylenchus dipsaci*).
1859	H Schacht	• First noticed cyst nematode of beet (*Heterodera schachtii*).
1931	NA Cobb	• Studied structure of many nematodes and classified them. • Coined the word nematology and developed many. techniques for the study of nematodes.
1892	Atkinson	• Reported that bacterial wilt of tomato was facilitated by root knot transmitted by nematode.
1958	Hewitt & Asso-ciates	• Discovered that the grape vine fan leaf virus was caused by nematode.
1958	Vasudeva	• Reported Molya disease of wheat (*Heterodera avenae*) from Rajasthan.
1961	Siddiqui	• Reported first time citrus nematode (*Tylenchulus semipenetrans*) from India. Reported potato cyst nematode for the first time from Nilgiri, India.
1961	Jones	• Reported that burrowing nematode on banana (*Radopholus similis*) for the first time from Kerala (India).
1970	Edward and Misra	• Incorporated root-knot nematode resistance, the Mi-1 gene, from the wild *Lycopersicon peruvianum* into the cultivated *L. esculentum* via embryo rescue
1994	PG Smith	• Suggested the use of nematodes as soil health indicators by testing an assay to check the soil ecosystem health by using the bacterial-feeding nematode (*Cruznema tripartitum*)
1997	SS Lau and Co workers	• Identified first nematode parasitism gene in the SVG cells of the cyst nematode.
1998	Smant and Co workers	• Identified first nematode gene encoding a signaling peptide from *Heterodera glycines.*

Year	Contributor (s)	Description
2001	Wang and Co workers	• Studied RNAi effects in plant parastic nematodes by using octopamine to stimulate oral ingestion by pre parasitic second-stage juveniles of cyst nematode (*H. glycines* and *G. pallida*).
2002	Urwin and Co workers	• Used predacious fungi to control plant-parasitic nematodes.
2002	Floyd and Co-workers	• Used DNA bar coding technique for the estimation of nematode diversity in Scottish grassland.
2005	Atibalentja and Co-workers	• Constructed first genetic map of *Heterodera glycines* and demostrated its utility by demonstrating mapping of Hg-Cm-1 gene.

Development of Plant Virology

Year	Contributor (s)	Description
1576	C Clusius	• Recorded breaking of tulips owing to viral infection.
1886	AE Mayer	• First to point out that tobacco mosaic is readily transmissible and infectious. • Demonstrated the sap transmission of the Tobacco mosaic virus.
1892	D Ivanowski	• Demonsrated that the agents of TMV could pass through filters that retained bacterial cells (bacteria proof filter).
1894	Hashimoto	• Showed transmissibility of rice dwarf disease by leaf hopper (*Nephotettix apicalis var. cincticeps*).
1898	MW Beijernick	• Concept of *contagium vivum fluidum* • He is known as Father of Plant Virology.
1917	d'Herelle	• Discovered bacteriophage
1931	Stahel	• Found flagellates (Protozoa) infecting the phloem of coffee trees, causing abnormal phloem formation and wilting of the trees.
1932	Knoll and Ruska	• Invented electron microscope.
1935	WM Stanley	• Crystallized Tobacco mosaic virus.
1936	F Bawden and NW Pirie	• Found that the crystalline nature of the virus • Viruses contains nucleic acid and protein.
1939	Kausche, Pfankuch and Ruska	• Initially observed viral particles with an electron microscope. • Confirmed that TMV was rod shaped.
1942 & 1944	Muller Williams and Wycoff	• Developed shadow casting technique with heavy metals which was useful for determining the overall size and shape of the virus particles.
1949	Markham and Smith	• Isolated Turnip yellow mosaic virus and showed that it contained (1) An infectious nucleoprotein (about 25%) and (2) non infectious protein.

Year	Contributor (s)	Description
1952	Morel and Martin	• Showed that virus free plants could be obtained from totally infected parents using meristem tip culture.
1954	Kassanis	• Showed that virus could be eradicated from infected plants by high temperature treatment.
1956	Gierer and Schramm	• Proved that the nucleic acid fraction of the virus is actually the infectious agent.
1966.	Kassanis	• Discovered the satellite viruses.
1963 & 1966	Black and Markhan; Miura and Co-workers	• Showed that wound tumour and rice dwarf viruses contain double started RNA.
1967	Doi and Co-workers	• Discovered Mycoplasma like organism.
1967	Ishiie and Co-workers	• Showed that the MLO bodies and the symptoms disappeared temporarily when the plants were treated with tetracycline antibodies.
1967	Diener and Raymer	• Discovered viroid.
1968	Shephard and Co-workers	• Showed that cauliflower mosaic virus contains double stranded DNA.
1974	Davies &Worley	• Coined the term spiroplasma.
1977	Clark and Adams	• Develpoed ELISA assay for detection of plant viruses.
1981	TW Randles and Co-workers	• Discovered virusoids.
1982	Prusiner	• Discovered Prions.
1994	Sears and Krikpatrick	• MLO that infects plants have been reclassified as Phytoplasmas.

Development of Genetics of Host Pathogen Interaction

Year	Contributor (s)	Description
1900-1909	Orton	• Working with wilt disease of cotton, watermelon and cowpea developed varieties that were resistant to the diseases. • Distinguished disease resistance from disease escape and disease endurance.
1905-1912	Biffen	• Described inheritance of resistance to yellow rust in two varieties of wheat and their progenies on the basis of Mendelian laws of inheritance.
1902	Ward	• Observed that colonization of resistant Bromus sp by *Puccinia dispersa* was accompanied by necrosis of the host cells adjacent to the colonizing fungus.
1903-04	Ward &Salmon	• Discovered physiologic specialization in fungi causing rust and powdery mildew of cereals.
1914	EC Stakman	• Reported that due to continuous evolution of races and biotypes in botanical species of the rust fungi, their physiologic capabilities go on changing in their favour, as a result of which the host plant resistance undergoes changes.

Year	Contributor (s)	Description
1915	Stakman	• Working on wheat *Puccinia graminis* system, also observed rapid cell death around the sites of penetration in resistant host plants and used the term hypersensitive to describe the response.
1940	Muller &Borger	• First identified phytoalexins as the antimicrobial compounds synthesized and accumulating at the site of infection or stress in plants , working on potato *Phytophthora infestans.*
1946	HF Flor	• Working with flax rust system, advance gene for gene hypothesis. • For every gene controlling resistance or susceptibility in the host, there must be matching genes for avirulence or virulence in the pathogen.
1963	Vanderplank	• Suggested that there are two kinds of resistance vertical (Major gene) and horizontal resistance (Minor gene).
1994	Erickson	• First discovered the phenomenon of variability among fungi. • Reported existence of physiologic races in the rust fungi.
1998	Gilchrist	• Reported possible connection between plant disease and programmed cell death, cell suicide or apoptosis associated with hypersensitive reaction.
1963	Cruickshank	• Confirmed accumulation of antimicrobial metabolites during pathological process and their role in resistance.

Development of Plant Disease Control

Year	Contributor (s)	Description
1000	Homer	• Mentioned about the use of sulphur in plant disease control.
Around 1200 A.D.	Albertus Magnus	• Mistletoe is the first plant pathogen to be recognized • First pathogen for which a cultural control (by pruning affected branches) was recommended.
1807	B Prevost	• Recommended copper sulphate for wheat seed treatment against bunt and demonstrated first time the fungitoxic value of copper compounds.
1882	PMA Millardet	• Discovered bordeaux mixture for control of downy mildew of grape vine.
1887	Mason	• Discovered burgundy mixture.
1921	Bewley	• Developed chestnut compound.
1934	Tisdale and Williams	• Reported fungitoxicity of dithiocarbamates.
1942	Singh	• Delveloped chaubatia paste.
1943	SA Waksman and A Schatx	• Discovered Streptomycin.
1952	Kittleson	• Discovered captan also known as Kittleson's Killer.
1966	Von Schmeling and M Kulka	• Discovered systemic fungicides oxanthin.

Development of Plant Pathology in India

Year	Contributor (s)	Description.
1885	KR Kritikar	• First Indian scientist who collected and identified fungi.
1886-1971	JF Dastur	• First Indian plant pathologist known for the etablishment of genus Phytophthora and diseases caused by it in castor and potato.
	TS Sadasivan	• Developed concept of vivotoxins and worked out the mechanism of wilting in cotton owing to *Fusarium oxysporum* f.sp. *vasinfectum*
	SN Dasgupta	• Carried out exensive study on black tip of mango.
	MJ Thrimalachar	• Discovered several antifungal antibiotics *viz* aureofungin, haymycin etc.
1960	YL Nene	• Reported khaira disease of rice caused due to Zn deficiency. • Authored book "Fungicides in Plant Disease Control."
1889	DD Cunningham	• Reported the causal organism of red rust of tea in Assam is *Cephaleurous virescens*
1920	EJ Butler	• First direcotor of Imperial Mycological Institue in England. • Initiated an exhaustive study on Indian fungi and the disease caused by them. • Discovered genus Allomyces. • Wrote "Fungi and Diseases in Plants". • He is known as Father of Indian Plant Pathology.
1940	KC Mehta	• Studied epidemiology of cereal rusts in India • Write monograph on "*Further studies on cereal rust in India*". • He is known as Father of Indian Rust.
1948	BB Mundukar	• Established Indian Phytopathological Society with its journal "*Indian Phytopathology*".
1953	JC Luthra and A Sattar	• Developed solar heat treatment for loose smut of wheat.
	Ramanujam and Co-workers	• Developed seed plot technique for virus free seed potato production in Indo Gangetic plains.
1975	S Nagrajan and H Singh	• Formulated Indian Stem Rust Rules for *Puccinia graminis tritici.*
	RS Singh	• Worked on biological control and ecology of soil borne pathogens. • His book Plant Diseases is referred as Bible of Plant Pathology.
	MM Payak	• Contributed significantly in maize pathology and multiple disease resistance.
	Ramanujam	• Develoed seed plot technique for virus free seed potato product ion in Indo gangetic plains.

4

Biotic and Abiotic Causes of Plant Diseases

Plant Pathogen

- Pathogen is an inducer of disease.
- A pathogen can therefore be defined as any factor that induces unresolved impairment or disruption of one or more important plant functions.
- Some plant functions such as nutrient uptake, are highly localized. Others, such as respiration, occur in all living tissues. Still others, such as photosynthesis and photorespiration, are extensively coordinated. Pathogen effects therefore range from very local to very general.
- Pathogens can cause disease in any one or many parts of a plant, from the smallest organelles and obscure metabolic pathways to entire cells, tissues, organs, and even entire plants.
- Some pathologists prefer to limit the term "pathogen" to living pathogens (they usually define it to include viruses and possibly viroids).
- However, diseases caused by abiotic factors (such as air pollutants and drought) have many similarities to diseases caused by biotic pathogens (such as toxigenic and wilt fungi). For this reason, we prefer to use the term "pathogen" to refer to any inducer of disease.
- When it is necessary to distinguish between live and non-living inducers, we use the terms "biotic" and "abiotic".
- Most biotic and many abiotic pathogens invade a host and cause disease. However, some pathogens exist only outside the host. They are called exopathogens (Woltz, 1978).
- Therefore, a pathogen may be defined as any biotic or abiotic factor that induces the sustained impairment of one or more vital processes in a plant or in any of its parts.

- Pathogens may act internally or externally, and we recognize that pathogens that interfere with coordinated use of energy pose a particularly serious threat to host health and survival.

A. Biotic Pathogens

- Biotic induces of disease are diverse.
- Fungi are the most common and they are the first pathogens to be studied in detail.
- Bacteria came after fungi, and shortly thereafter nematodes were shown to cause disease in plants.
- More recently, viruses, viroids and plasmids, mycoplasma and rickettsia etc have been added.
- Mistletoe was recognized as a plant parasite long before fungi but the idea that mistletoe is also a pathogen is only 40 years old.
- Many parasitic and pathogenic seed plants are now recognized.
- Chemical warfare (allelopathy) in higher plants is a new dimension in plant pathology.
- Some insects (such as grasshoppers and caterpillars) damage plants, while others carry plant pathogens.
- However, many insects are pathogens themselves.
- They cause disease in the same spirit as nematodes, fungi and bacteria!.
- Gall-forming insects cause abnormal growth.
- Mites, reed turtles and webworms interfere with photosynthesis. They induce chlorosis and necrosis of leaf and stem tissues.
- Woodworms disrupt xylem function and impair the supply of nutrients and water to stems and leaves.
- Aphids, scale insects, and thrips cause cell damage.
- Bark beetles, weevils, nematodes, and larvae interfere with food and water transport in stems and roots.
- Seed and cone insects interfere with reproduction.
- Certain weevils attack flowering parts or kill young seedlings.

Why insects are not recognized as plant pathogens.

- In many countries, entomology is considered a separate discipline from plant pathology.
- This pattern of biologist declustering has suppressed interaction between pathologists and entomologists for decades.
- Most plant pathologists are botanists and are primarily interested in the biology of plant hosts, while entomologists are zoologists and are primarily interested in the biology of insects.
- Whatever the overall reason for the reluctance, we believe the time has come to change the attitudes of both plant pathologists and entomologists towards insects and their role in plant disease.
- A collaboration between scholars in these two fields offers great potential for mutually productive research.
- Insects that cause persistent disruption of vital plant functions are pathogens .

B. Viruses, Viroids and Plasmids

- Some plant pathologists include viruses, viroids, and plasmids among biotic pathogens.
- Others consider them abiotic pathogens.
- Some people do not consider plasmids to be pathogens at all.
- However, the biochemical properties, reproductive modalities, and pathogenic mechanisms of all three entities are so similar and so unique that they should be placed in their own class.
- Viruses contain two main parts, a nucleic acid core and a protein coat.
- Viroids are particles of naked nucleic acid. They lack a protein shell.
- Plasmids (and episomes) are extrachromosomal pieces of DNA found in bacterial cells.
- Recently, a plasmid of *Agrobacterium tumafacians* was shown to be responsible for the ability of this bacterium to induce tumors in plants.
- A plasmid containing an "oncogenic code" can apparently be transferred into the cells of a plant host by bacteria.

- These two observations lead to the conclusion that plasmids are pathogens and their bacterial hosts are vectors .
- Similar observations of cytoplasmic transmissible factors that regulate virulence in Helminthosporium and Endothia suggest that viruses, viroids, plasmids, and episomes can affect plants and pathogenic microorganisms. suggest that it may represent part of a continuum of particles inhabiting .
- Each plays an important and characteristic role in plant disease.
- All of these entities contain nucleic acids. They all lack their own metabolic capacity.
- They all reproduce and cause disease by redirecting part of the host cell's metabolic machinery to synthesize viruses, viroids, plasmids, or episomal particles in place of host nucleic acids and proteins.
- Neither biotic nor abiotic pathogens can do that! Viruses, viroids, and plasmids are truly unique,

Table 3: Comparison between different plant pathogens

Features	Fungi	Bacteria	Viruses	Viroids	Phytoplasma	Sprioplasma	RLO	Protozoa	Algae	Nematode
Visibility in micorscope	Yes	Yes	No (visible under Electronmic-roscope)	No (visible under Electron microscope)	Yes	Yes	Yes	Yes	Yes	Yes
Prokaryote / Eukaryote	Eukaryote	Prokaryote	Kingdom -Virus	-	Prokaryote	Prokaryote	Prokaryote	Eukaryote	Eukaryote	Eukaryote
Cell Wall	Present	Present	Absent	Absent	Absent	Absent	Present	Present	Present	Present
Cell wall with mucopoly saccharides	No	Yes	Yes	No	No	No	Yes	No	No	No
Nucleic acid	Both DNA & RNA	Both DNA & RNA	Either DNA & RNA	RNA	Both DNA & RNA	Both DNA & RNA	Both DNA & RNA	Both DNA & RNA	Both DNA & RNA	Both DNA & RNA
Protein synthesis by their own enzyme	Yes	Yes	No	No	Yes	Yes		Yes	Yes	Yes
Culture in cell free medium	Yes	Yes	Yes	No	No	No	Xylem inhibitory fastidious vascular bacteria can be cultured	Yes	Yes	Yes
Dependent on host nucleic acid for multiplication	No	No		No	No	No	No	No	No	No
Reproduction	Asexual &Sexual	Binary fission	Replication	Replication	Binary fission	Binary fission	Binary fission	Asexual &Sexual	Asexual &Sexual	Asexual &Sexual

Examples of biotic causes of plant diseases

- **Fungi** e.g. Wilt of cotton,Black rust of wheat,Late blight of potato
- **Bacteria** e.g. Citrus canker, Bacterial blight of rice, Angular leaf spot of cotton
- **Rickettsia-like bacteria** (RLB) e.g. Citrus greening, Pierce's disease of grape
- **Viruses** e.g. Yellow mosaic of blackgram, Soybean mosaic, Tomato leaf curl
- **Viroids** e.g. Spindle tuber of potato
- **Mycoplasma-like organism (MLO)** e.g. Sesame phyllody, Little leaf of egg plants
- **Spiroplasma** e.g. Corn stunt, Citrus stubborn
- **Protozoa** e.g. Heart rot of coconut
- **Algae** e.g. Red rust of mango
- **Nematodes** –Root knot nematode, Golden nematode, Seed gall nematode

C. Abiotic Pathogens

Definition

Plant disease in which no pathogens or parasitic is associate with the cause is known as Non-parasitic disease. They are also called as non-infectious or physiological disorders.

General Characteristics

Factors causative of physiological disorders

1. Effect of temperature

i) Effects of low temperatures

1. It does more damage to plants than high temperatures.
2. Frost damage includes the death of peaches, cherry buds, flowers, young fruits and sometimes the juicy branches of most trees.
3. Cold winter temperatures can kill the young roots of trees such as apples, causing cankers and splitting of the bark.

ii) Effects of high temperature

1. Plants usually get hurt quickly.
1. Responsible for sun damage occurring on the sun-exposed side of fleshy fruits and vegetables. for example. tanned apples, tomatoes, onions, peppers, potato tubers and flaxseed shrimp.

2. Effect of humidity

(i). Effects of low humidity

1. Plants generally remain stunted.
2. Light green to light yellow leaves,
3. Let dry and wilt.

ii) Effects of high humidity

1. The fibrous roots of plants rot and wilt.
2. Toxic substances build up around roots and stem bases.
3. Nutrients are not available. For example. Tip burn by paddy.

3. Effect of low oxygen

1. Destruction of cells by enzymatic action. For example. Black heart of potato.

4. Effect of unfavorable light

1. Slows down the formation of chlorophyll.
2. Internodes are long and elongated
3. Light green leaves, spiral habit, premature leaf and flower drop. This state is called "Etiolation".

5. Effect of air pollution

1. The presence of harmful gases in the atmosphere can cause obvious damage to equipment.
2. Chemicals such as hydrogen fluoride, nitrogen dioxide, ozone, sulfur dioxide and peroxyacothyl nitrate cause more severe and widespread damage to field crops. For example. black tip of mango.
3. Fruit from trees near brickyards may exhibit necrotic lesions, making them unsuitable for sale or consumption.

4. Smoke from brick kiln polluted the air with toxic gases such as sulfur dioxide-like gases that cause tissue necrosis.

6. Toxicity of soil minerals and toxic effects of decomposition of organic matters in soil

1. Excessive amounts of sodium salts, especially sodium sulfate, sodium chloride, and sodium carbonate, increase soil pH and cause alkali damage. Ex. Chlorosis, etc.
2. Boron, copper, and manganese are often associated with mineral poisoning diseases.
3. Excess manganese is known to cause wrinkle leaf disease in cotton.
4. Excess boron is toxic to many vegetables and trees.
5. Crop residues that decompose in the soil produce toxic substances such as fatty acids that cause wilt, root rot, and symptoms of nutritional deficiencies.

7. Herbicide damage

1. Some of the most common plant diseases appear to be the result of widespread herbicide use.
2. The growing number of herbicides used for general or specific weed control poses a problem.

8. Nutritional deficiencies or disorder in plants

1. Deficiency of minerals *viz, nitrogen, phosphorus, potash, manganese , zinc, copper, iron, magnesium, boron,* etc. results in disorders in plant metabolism and cause *hunger signs* in the crops
2. Excess and deficiency of minerals disturbs nutritional balance needed for good metabolism in the plant, hence hindering the effect of essential element.
3. The deficiencies and excess of minerals also reduce the resistance of plant to fungal, bacterial and other diseases.
4. The kind of symptoms produced by deficiency of a certain nutrient depend primarily on the functions of that particular element in the plant.
5. Nutrient mobility plays an important role in determining the site of the deficiency symptoms.

6. For *highly mobile* elements like *nitrogen and potassium*, the deficiency symptoms appear predominantly in *older* and mature leaves.
7. Deficiency of *poorly mobile* elements, like *calcium, boron* and *iron* show up in *younger* leaves.
8. The symptoms of deficiency of *moderately mobile* elements like *magnesium* and *sulphur,* are uniformly spread all over the plant.
9. The symptoms of mineral deficiencies is recorded in the following table:

Sr.No	**Deficient element**	**Symptoms**
1	Nitrogen	Poor growth, chlorosis of leaves, delayed flowering and fruiting.
2	Phosphorus	Poor growth, blue/green, but not yellow colour of leaves, oldest leaves affected first.
3	Potassium	Brown scorching and curling of leaf tip, yellowing of leaf veins.
4	Calcium	Curling and tip burn of leaves, stunted growth, abnormal development of meristmatic tissues, and eventual death of buds and root tips. Also causes bitter pit in apple.
5	Magnesium	Interveinal chlorosis, giving a mottled appearance to leaves similar to virus infection.
6	Sulfur	Chlorotic leaves, petioles and veins distinctly red.
7	Iron	Chlorosis of leaves, young leaves appear bleached, symptoms similar to manganese deficiency.
8	Manganese	Chlorotic leaves with green veins.
9	Zinc	Younger leaves yellow, pitting on lower leaf surface, leaves and internodes shortened, giving a rosette-like look to plants; guttation increased.
10	Copper	Leaves pale and curled; petioles droop down.
11	Boron	Drying of growing tip, bushy stunted growth, and internal tissue breakdown.
12	Molybdenum	Chlorosis of leaves; symptoms similar to nitrogen deficiency. Also causes whiptail disease in cauliflower.

Table : Plant disease due to lack of minerals

Sr.No	Deficient Nutrient	Disease
1	Nitrogen (N)	Red leaf of cotton
2	Phosphorus (P)	Dwarfening of cotton
3	Potassium (K)	Cotton rust leaf spot of alfa alfa.
4	Magnesium (Mg)	Sand drown disease in tobacco

5	Boron (B)	Internal cork of apple Cracked stem of celery Black tip of mango Heart rot of sugarbeet Brown heart of cabbage and turnip Internal brown spot of sweet potato Terminal bud breakdown of tobacco Fruit pitting and dieback of olive Hollow stem of brassica
6	Copper (Cu)	Reclamation disease of oats Diebacks of citrus Wither tip of apple
7	Manganese (Mn)	Pahala blight of sugarcane Marsh spot of garden pea Grey speck of oats.
8	Zinc (Zn)	White bud of corn Little leaf of apple Bronzing of twigs Rosette of fruits trees Mottle leaf of citrus Khaira disease of rice
9	Iron (Fe)	Green netting of citrus
10	Molybdenum (Mo)	Whiptail disease of cauliflower
11	Calcium(Ca)	Blossom end rot of tomato Black heart of celery Wither tip of flax

D. Distinguish between hungry parasites and irritant pathogens

- Nature has evolved a magnificent series of relationships and interactions between organisms.
- This array represents a continuum that is difficult to grasp as a whole.
- To better understand these complex relationships, scientists have found it helpful to categorize things.
- Essentially, we divide the natural continuum into components and divisions.
- Components and divisions are sufficiently similar in substance and sufficiently different in substance that an understanding of the whole is more easily achieved.
- This process is sometimes called pigeonholding.
- Pigeonholding is a well-developed technique in plant pathology.

- Four particular sets of pigeonholes have proven to be very useful in plant pathology.
- They include his four sets of concepts:
  - Mutualism, Commensalism, Pathosism, Saprophytism
  - Predators, Pathogens, Parasites, Perthophyte, Saprophytes
  - Obligate parasites, Facultative saprophytes, Facultative parasites, Obligate saprophytes.
  - Obligatory biotrophism, Facultative necrotrophism, Facultative biotrophism, Obligate necrotrophism .
- Horsfall and Dimond (1960), proposed the famous "mother-in-law analogy" to explain the essential difference between parasites and pathogens.
- They used the terms 'hungry parasite' and 'irritating pathogen'.
- Parasitism is a process by which energy and substance for growth and development of parasite are obtained at the expense of the host.
- Thus the terms 'hungry parasite' and 'nourishing host' make for a useful description of host parasitic relationships.
- Pathogenesis is the process by which critical plant functions are impaired or disrupted by the continued stimulation of pathogens.
- Again, the terms 'stimulant' and 'affected' or 'disturbed host' provide useful descriptions of reality.
- It is clear that not all parasites are pathogens and not all pathogens are parasites.
- Pathogens can be biotic or abiotic.
- Biotic pathogens can be parasitic or non-parasitic.
- A susceptible organism is called a suscept and may or may not be a host.
- The term suscept is useful because pathogens may not be parasites.
- So we have the host-parasite and suspect-pathogen couplets.
- A host-pathogen pair is correct only if the pathogen is a parasite.
- In all cases involving disease, the couplet susceptibility pathogen is correct and has a specific meaning.

5

Growth and Reproduction of Plant Pathogen

1. Growth of plant pathogens

Various plant pathogens, namely fungi, bacteria, nematodes, viruses, viroids, mollicutes, fastidious bacteria, and protozoa, grow in different ways.

1.1 Fungi and parasitic higher plants

- Fungal pathogens and parasitic higher plants usually invade and infect tissues by growing on or in them from the first point of inoculation.
- Most of these pathogens, whether they cause small lesions or large infected areas on the plant, grow, branch, and spread to more and more plant tissues until the infection stops spreading or the plant dies.
- Fungi that cause vascular wilting often enter plants by producing and releasing spores within vessels, which, when carried in the sap stream, enter vessels distant from the mycelium and germinate. to generate and invade other vessels.

1.2. Other plant pathogens

- Bacteria, mollicutes, viruses, viroids, nematodes, and protozoa do not increase in size over time.
- Their size and shape remain relatively unchanged throughout their existence.
- These pathogens invade and infect new tissues within the plant and multiply rapidly in infected tissues to greatly increase their numbers.
- The progeny are then passively transported to new cells and tissues.
    - Plasmids: viruses and viroids.
    - Phloem: viruses, viroids, mollicutes, some pathogenic bacteria, protozoa.
    - Xylem: some bacteria, protozoa, nematodes.

2. Pathogen Reproduction

Various plant pathogens, namely fungi, bacteria, nematodes, viruses, viroids, mollicutes, fastidious bacteria and protozoa reproduce in different ways.

2.1. Fungi

- Fungi use spores to reproduce. Spores are either asexual (fission spores, i.e. products of mitosis) or sexual (meiosis spores, i.e. products of meiosis).
- Most phytopathogenic fungi and oomycetes produce mycelia only within the infected plant and produce spores on or just below the surface of the host's infected area, which are released into the environment.
- Few fungi or oomycetes produce mycelium on the surface of the host plant, but most powdery mildew produce mycelium only on the surface of the host plant and not inside the host plant. The clubroot pathogens and fungi that cause vascular wilt produce spores within the host tissue that are not released until the host dies and disperses.
- Some fungi produce spores more or less continuously, while others produce continuously by maturity. Either way, hundreds to thousands of spores can be produced per square centimeter of infected tissue.
- Even small, specialized sporophytes can produce millions of spores, often billions or trillions of spores produced per diseased plant.
- Therefore, the number of spores produced by one hectare of heavily infected crops is generally astronomical and sufficient spores are released to reach the surface of a conceivable field and surrounding areas.

2.2. Bacteria

- The bacterium reproduces by fission in which a mature individual divides into her two equal smaller individuals.
- Bacteria multiply within host cells, usually within host plants, among bacteria that live in the xylem or phloem.
- They only reach the surface of the host through wounds, cracks, and stomata.
- Bacteria multiply rapidly in infected tissue.
- Under optimal nutritional and environmental conditions (during culture), bacteria divide (double in number) every 20-30 minutes, and bacteria in

susceptible plants will as long as it is, it will probably grow at the same rate.

- A single drop of infected plant sap can contain millions of bacteria, so the number of bacteria per plant must be large.

2.3. Viruses and Viroids

- Viruses and viroids replicate only within cells and do not appear to reach or reside on the surface of the host plant.
- Just as pages placed on a copier are duplicated by the machine, they are duplicated by the cell as long as the machine is running and the paper supply continues.
- They multiply in live host cells and the first new virus particles are detected hours after infection.
- However, as soon as virus particles accumulate inside infected living cells, there can be up to 100,000-10,000,000 particles in a single cell.
- Viruses and viroids infect and multiply in most or all of the host's living cells. It is clear that any plant can contain myriad individuals of these pathogens.

2.4. Fastidious bacteria and Mollicutes and Protozoa

- Mollicutes, protozoa, and fastidious bacteria reproduce only intracellularly and do not appear to reach or be present on the surface of the host plant.
- Stubborn bacteria and mollicutes also reproduce by division. In this division, the mature individual divides into her two equal smaller individuals.
- Troublesome bacteria and mollicutes seem to grow more slowly than typical bacteria. Although they are systemically distributed throughout the vasculature of plants.
- They are present in relatively few xylem or phloem vessels, and the total number of these pathogens in infected plants is relatively low.
- This also seems to apply to protozoa.

2.5. Nematodes

- Nematodes reproduce through eggs.
- Female nematodes lay 300 to 500 eggs, nearly half of which produce females that again lay 300 to 600 eggs each.
- A nematode species can have from 2 generations to 10 or more generations per year, depending on climate, host availability, and the length of each nematode's life cycle.
- If even half the female survives and reproduces, each generation increases the number of nematodes in the soil by more than 100 times.
- Therefore, increases in nematode populations during the growing season and subsequent seasons are often very dramatic.

6

Survival and Dispersal of Important Plant Pathogens

Plant diseases are a recurring threat. Everywhere they appear in a certain cycle. Chains of infection (pathogenesis) initiated by primary inoculums comes spontaneously at the end of the harvest season or at host death due to the production of various types of pathogenic reproductive organs/propagules. These propagules must find ways to bridge the gap between harvest times to ensure continuity of infection. Therefore, plant pathogen survival is a critical step in a successful pathogen disease cycle. Pathogen spread is another important phenomenon in plant disease recurrence and epidemiology. Effective spread/diffusion of virulent propagules is critical for initiation of chains of infection and further progression of the disease in time and space.

Thus, two key aspects of any plant disease cycle are (i) how pathogens survive during the growing season or periods of adverse environmental conditions, and (ii) how one diseased plant infects another. Disease does not occur if survival or spread is prevented. Therefore, knowledge of survival and spread mechanisms often reveals weak links in the disease cycle that can be used to control or manage the disease.

1. Survival of Plant Pathogens

The availability of plant pathogens in a given area depends not only on their ability to survive during parasitic relationships with their hosts, but also on their ability to survive in seasons when the hosts are not growing. The part that remains quiescent to overcome the unfavorable host unavailability is called 'survival'. Pathogens develop by acting as saprophytes in specialized dormant structures, in or on the soil, or in diseased plant debris, or by living in close association with living plants and other organisms. Means of survival are the first link in the chain of infection or the cycle of disease. The first infection that arises from a viable source of pathogens in culture is the primary infection, and the organ of transmission that causes this infection is called the primary inoculum. After a disease outbreak in a crop, spores or other structures of the pathogen serve as a secondary inoculum, causing secondary infection and thereby spreading the disease in the field. Most plant pathogens can only survive by repeatedly reinfecting the host plant. This process of repeated infection is called the infection chain. If the chain of infection is broken, the pathogen dies. Chains of infection can be divided into two types based on how the pathogen inoculum survives from leaving an infected host (distributor host) to reaching an infecting host (recipient host).

1.1 Continuous chains of infection: In continuous chains of infection, pathogens survive by continuously infecting susceptible plants without interruption.

(1.1.1). Continuous chain of infection by the same host or another host.

(1.1.2). Continuous chain of infection by alternative hosts.

1.2. Discontinuous chains of infection: Discontinuous chains of infection exist when the disease cycle is interrupted by epiphytic, saprophytic, or stationary phases.

(1.2.1) Discontinuous chain of infection with resting phase.

(1.2.2). Discontinuous chain of infection with epiphytic phase.

(1.2.3). Discontinuous chain of infection with a saprophytic phase.

1.1 Continuous chains of infection

1.1.1 Continuous chain of infection by the same host or another host

- A continuous chain of infection by the same or different hosts occurs when the parasite survives by continuously infecting plants of the same host species or different plant species than the main crop species.
- Such plants are called alternative hosts and are often associated with crop species.
- If the alternate host, often a weedy species, does not show disease symptoms, it is called a disease vector.
- Parasites do not form dormant structures and do not live saprophytically or epiphytically on plant surfaces.
- Survival therefore depends on the presence of susceptible host plants. Such chains of infection are common to all major groups of plant pathogens.

- In addition to crops, some undesirable plants (such as weeds) grow independently in nature, both annuals and perennials. Plants belonging to the same plant family to which the cultured host belongs are called collateral hosts/alternative hosts.
- An example is the survival of three Puccinia species causes wheat rust on the Indian subcontinent. These fungi survive the active sporulation stage of wild species of Triticum, Aegilops, Horedeum, and Agropyron repens.
- Similarly, rice tungro viruses live actively in the genera Oryza and Echinochloa. and *Leersia hexandra*
- Parasitic organisms on perennials (fruit trees, plantations, forest trees) live either actively or passively in or on the host, depending on environmental conditions.
- Certain pathogens, namely *X. compestris pv citri*, *X. compestris pv jugalandis*, *X. compestris pv. pruni* and *Erwinia amylovora* are known to be constantly transmitted by residues or rotten twigs, and can produce bacterial sludge on fresh inoculum in good weather.
- Similarly, some fungal plant pathogens such as *Colletotrichum gloeosporioides* (anthracnose of mango), *Oidium mangiferae* (powdery mildew of mango) and *Podosphaera leucotricha* (powdery mildew of apple) survive on infected plant organs.

1.1.2 Continuous infection chains involving alternate hosts

- Some plant pathogens are not directly transmitted from an infected plant to another plant of the same species.
- They must switch between her two completely unrelated species.
- Some heterocious rust fungi require another host for the infection chain.
- Example: The heterocyst fungus requires two of her host plants, wheat and barberry, to complete her life cycle. Other hosts do not belong to the plant family of cultured hosts and are offered as alternate hosts.
- The disease cycle cannot be completed without an alternate host.
- Even with the most advanced technology available today, scientists cannot directly transmit most plant viruses and phytoplasmas from one plant to another.

- They are transmitted only through vectors (usually, but not always, insects).
- Viruses often enter into a biological relationship with a vector and replicate partially within the vector.
- The vector thus functions as an alternative or intermediate host, and the chain of infection alternates between her two unrelated species. The chain of infection is therefore plant-insect-vector-plant. If no alternative host (vector) is found, the chain of infection is broken.

1.2. Discontinuous chains of infection:

1.2.1. Discontinuous infection chains involving a resting stage

- Some plant pathogens are not directly transmitted from an infected plant to another plant of the same species.
- Must switch between two completely independent species.
- Some heterologous rust fungi require additional hosts for infection chains.
- Example: A heterocyst fungus requires her two host plants of wheat and barberry to complete its life-her cycle. Other hosts do not belong to the plant family of cultured hosts and serve as alternative hosts.
- A disease cycle cannot be completed without an alternative host.
- Using the most advanced technology currently available, scientists cannot directly transmit most plant viruses and phytoplasmas from one plant to another.
- They are transmitted only by vectors (usually, but not always, insects).
- Viruses often enter into a biological relationship with a vector and replicate partially within the vector. The vector thus acts as an alternative or intermediate host, and the chain of infection alternates between its two unrelated species. The infection chain is therefore plant-insect-vector-plant. If no alternative host (vector) is found, the chain of infection is interrupted.

1.2.2. Discontinuous infection chains involving an epiphytic phase

- Some fungal and bacterial pathogens live on the surfaces of hosts and other plants in a non-parasitic relationship as epiphytes.

- For example, the peach leaf curly fungus (*Taphrina deformans*) develops yellow to reddish areas on the leaves that gradually thicken and curl, causing the leaves to curl and fall prematurely.
- Naked asci containing ascospores form on the upper surface of the wavy leaves.
- Ascospores germinate to form budding yeast-like conidia that can only infect very young leaves that are not available at the time the budding colony is formed.
- The fungus grows as epiphytes on the bark and scales of the next year's leaf buds during the summer (when only mature leaves are present on the tree) and during the winter (when no leaves are present on deciduous peach trees).
- The following spring, when the leaf buds swell and the young leaves begin to grow, budding cells infect the young leaves and form a mycelium in the undifferentiated young host tissue.
- Fungi form asci in early summer and complete their life cycle. A single application of fungicide (such as a copper-based spray) by him just before spring budding is sufficient to control peach leaf curl.

- Bacterial apical necrosis caused by *Pseudomonas syringae pv. syringae* cause sunken rot in the woody tissue of affected trees, often exuding gum. Infection can lead to premature death of the entire tree or infected branches.
- Bacteria overwinter in crustaceans, multiply in spring, and spread on leaves by rain spray, where they develop large epiphytic communities.
- These epiphytes become the main source of inoculum for wound and leaf stigma infection the following fall.
- The same bacteria also cause pea rot.
- Again, bacteria are present as part of the normal flora on the surface of healthy pea leaves. Infection occurs after injuring the plant.

1.2.3. Discontinuous infection chains involving a saprophytic phase

- Many fungi and phytopathogenic bacteria survive as saprophytes on diseased plant debris and organic matter present in or on the soil during cover crops.
- For example, apple scab (*Venturia inaequalis*) attack apple leaves and fruit in spring and summer.

    - The fungus overwinters as the initials on infected leaves and berries that fall to the ground in autumn.
    - After the mycelium of the suitable mating type coalesces in autumn, a black tentacle occurs on fallen leaves.
    - The fungus then overwinters in fallen leaves. The following spring, pseudotesia produce ascospores that serve as the primary inoculum to start the disease cycle in the new season.
    - Primary infection by ascospore infection produces conidia that serve as a secondary inoculum that contributes to the development of epidemics.
- Pathogens that can survive in or on the soil by saprophytic growth are generally classified into her two types: soil dwellers and soil invaders.
- Soil dwellers are facultative parasites that can survive indefinitely in soil as saprophytes and have a variety of hosts. Pythium, Rhizoctonia, and Fusarium are good examples of soil-dwelling fungal pathogens.
- Soil invaders (soil fugitives) are more specialized parasites that generally live in close association with their hosts, but are able to survive in soil for relatively short periods of time as saprophytes.
- Most facultative saprophytic bacterial and fungal pathogens are soil invaders.

• Differentiate Soil inhabitants and soil invaders

Sl.No	Soil inhabitants	Soil invaders / Root inhabiting fungi
1	Unspecialized parasites with a wide host range that are able to survive in soils indefinitely as saprophytes.	Specialized parasites that survive in soils in close association with their hosts.
2	Include obligate saprophytes and facultative parasites which are exo-pathogens	Include facultative saprophytes which are endopathogens (root infecting fungi).
3	Soil and plant debris serve as media for their saprophytic survival.	The active saprophytic phase remains as long as the host tissue in which they were living as parasites is not completely decomposed.
4	High competitive saprophytic survival ability.	Low competitive saprophytic survival ability.

Sl.No	Soil inhabitants	Soil invaders / Root inhabiting fungi
5	Plant pathogenic bacteria {e.g. *Agrobacterium rhizogenes* which causes crown gall, *Ralstonia solanacearum* which causes bacterial wilt and *Streptomyces scabies* which causes common scab of potato) and fungi (e.g. damping-off fungi and several species of Fusarium, Pythium and Rhizoctonia) can compete very effectively as saprophytes with the normal soil microflora. These parasites are often referred to as *soil inhabitants* because they are part of the normal soil microflora.	Vascular wilt causing species of *Fusarium, Verticillium* and take-all fungus of wheat (*Gaeumannomyces graminis var. tritici*) etc., are soil invaders.

1.3. Survival through insects

- Survival of plant pathogens associated with insects is not uncommon in nature.
- Some vectors, such as aphids and ticks, carry non-persistent viruses externally or near mouthparts.
- Viruses are known to contaminate crops within vectors that are themselves dormant. In persistent viruses, on the other hand, the vector remains infectious for much longer, sometimes for life, or the infectivity is passed on to the next generation.
- This allows the virus to manage the continuity of its infection cycle.
- Barley yellow mosaic virus can survive for up to 10 years in dormant spores of its vector (*Polymyxa gramins*), and tobacco rattle virus for approximately 1 year in dormant nematodes.
- The bacterium associated with maize wilt (*E. stewartii*) is present in the gut of the vector.
- Nematodes play a key role in the survival and spread of many important plant viruses.

1.4. Nematode survival

- At least 20 plant viruses are known to be perennial along with soil-dwelling ectoparasitic nematodes.
- Nematodes of the genera Longidorus and Xiphinema acquire viral pathogens such as tobacco ring-spot, tomato ring-spot, tomato and wheat spindle stripe mosaic, and nematodes of the genera Trichodorus and Paratrichodorus acquire diseases such as ringworm of tobacco and peas.

1.5.Survival by fungi

- Some viral pathogens have been found to survive in association with certain fungi.
- Olpidium is the source of survival and transmission of the viral pathogens responsible for tobacco mosaic, cucumber necrosis, lettuce, and tobacco stunting.
- The viruses that cause wheat mosaic disease and necrotic grapevine disease in beets survive in his one fungus, Polymyxa, while the virus that causes moptop disease in potatoes survives in Spongosproa.
- These viruses are carried internally or externally by dormant spores and zoospores of their respective fungi.
- Such dormant spores and zoospores introduce the virus into the host plant when the virus infects the host plant.

2. Dispersal of Pathogens

To make a healthy plant sick or diseased, a pathogen's primary requirement is to spread its inoculum from a surviving source to susceptible hosts. The spread in is called spread. Both centimeters of inoculum displacement and hundreds of kilometers of transport represent its spread. However, pathogen spread does not necessarily only help spread the disease, it also helps continue the pathogen life cycle and development. An accurate understanding of pathogen spread is necessary to find effective disease control measures. Because there is always a way to prevent the spread and break the chain of infection.

Plant pathogen dispersal generally occurs through two key groups:

2.1. Direct (Autonomous) dispersal: - The pathogen is carried through

2.1.1. Soil

2.1.2. Seed

2.1.3. Planting material

2.2. Indirect (Passive) dispersal:- The pathogen spreading itself or by natural agencies like

2.2.1. Wind

2.2.2. Water

2.2.3. Animals

2.2.4. Insects

2.2.5. Mites

2.2.6. Nematodes

2.2.7. Birds

2.1. Direct (Autonomous) dispersal

2.1.1. Through the soil: Numerous plant pathogens survive in the soil. Their survival in soil depends on many factors, including soil properties, soil environment, crops being grown, and other agricultural practices. In soil it spreads in two ways

a. Dissemination in soil (when the soil remains stationary but the pathogen grows or moves). Many pathogens survive in soil as facultative parasites or saprophytes. Some fungi produce motile spores (zoospores) that travel to some extent in the soil and infect the host. The nematode travels to some extent in the soil and infects the host.

b. Dissemination through soil – Contaminated soil is transported to other locations using agricultural practices, such as planting material, seedlings, or equipment.

2.1.2. Through the seed: Infected/affected seeds are one of the most important means of autonomous spread. Dissemination of the inoculum by seeds occurs as follows.

- Dormant structures of pathogen mixtures and contaminants ex. galls, sclerotia, cysts, smut. Example: Jowar's smut is an example of the former type and the fungal structure is called "Sclerotia" of bajra ergot.
- By the presence of propagules on the seed coat.
- As a dormant mycelium in seeds, e.g. loose smut of wheat, ring rot and brown rot of potatoes, whip smut and red rot of sugarcane, mosaic and leaf rot of potatoes.

2.1.3. Through vegetative planting materials: The spread of many plant pathogens occurs through the vegetative parts of plants used as planting material like tubers, cuttings, runners, rhizomes, grafts, etc. More than 40% of bacterial plant pathogens are transmitted by vegetatively propagated material. Important examples include *X. compestris pv.citri* (citrus canker) and *A. tumifaciens* (crown gall). Viruses are always transmitted by vegetative propagules. Viral diseases are therefore serious mainly in vegetatively propagated horticultural crops.

Table : Autonomous dispersal of plant pathogens

Autonomous dispersal	Examples
Through seed	
Seed contamination	*Anguina tritici* (Seed gall nematode), *Tolyposporium penicillariae* (Smut of bajra), Claviceps , Cuscuta
Internally seed borne	Loose smut of wheat *(Ustilago tritici)*
Externally seed borne	Covered smut of barley (*Ustilago hordei*), Stinging smut of wheat (*Tilletia caries* and *Tilletia foetida),* Black arm of cotton *(Xanthomonas campestris* pv. *mavacearum)*
Through vegetative planting materials	
Seed tubers	Late blight of potato (*Phytophthora infestans*)
Sugarcane Sets/cutting	Red rot of sugarcane(*Colletotrichum falcatum*)
Propagative materials	Citrus tristeza and Greening
Rhizome	Rhizome rot of ginger

2.2. Indirect (Passive) dispersal

2.2.1. Wind dispersal: - Fungal spores produced exogenously on the surface of the host are most easily carried by wind currents. Widespread and severe epidemics of plant diseases are usually the result of wind-driven spread of pathogens. Wind dispersal has four stages associated with spores. Infection is triggered under favorable climatic conditions by production of numerous spores, release into wind currents, wind dispersal, and deposition on surfaces of new susceptible hosts. This is the most dangerous transmission route for plant pathogens such as powdery mildew, downy mildew, leaf spot, blight and rust.

2.2.2. Water dispersal: The spread of diseases by various methods through water is relatively minor compared to wind spread. Flying raindrops commonly transmit leaf diseases from leaf to leaf, shoot to shoot, and even plant to plant in dense crops. Plant pathogens that require high humidity conditions, such as downy mildew-causing fungi and citrus canker-causing bacteria, are well adapted to this short-range water dispersion mode. Certain soil-dwelling pathogenic fungi and bacteria that cause root rot, blight, and foot rot can be transmitted over much greater distances through irrigation water, streams, and rivers. It also plays an important role in seed transmission from higher flowering parasites such as dodder and striga.

2.2.3. Insect dispersal: Most viral plant diseases are transmitted by a variety of insects. Viral diseases can be transmitted by sucking, chewing, or biting insects. Transmission is simply “mechanical” or “biological”. In mechanical transmission, pathogens are simply carried outward or inward by insects. In biology, there is some connection or relationship between certain insects and certain viral pathogens. In such cases, the insect is called the "vector" of the respective viral pathogen. There are two types of viruses that are "biologically" transmitted by insect vectors:

2.2.3.1. Non-persistent ;Viral pathogens that do not require latent period or incubation period within the insect.

2.2.3.2. Persistence: A viral pathogen that requires a certain incubation period within the vector body before inoculation or transfer to a healthy host. Insects involved in transmitting viral diseases belong to species such as aphids, jacids, whiteflies and mealybugs. Certain bacteria, namely potato fire (*E. amylovora*), citrus canker (*X. citri*), and some fungal pathogens, namely *Ceratostomella ulmi*, cucumber anthracnose (*Colletotrichum lagenarium*), are also transmitted by insects known to be contagious.

2.2.3.2.1. Mites dispersal: Mites are the only non-insect arthropod vectors of plant viruses. The ability to transmit viruses is limited to some species of ticks. Diseases transmitted by freeze-dried mites include fig mosaic, pigeon pea sterile mosaic, wheat streak mosaic and wheat blotch mosaic.

2.2.3.2.2 Nematodes dispersal: Nematodes have been observed to carry viral, bacterial, and fungal plant diseases. Nematodes that externally feed on host plant roots damage the roots and become an entry route for fungal and bacterial pathogens that infect plant roots. Members of the genera Longidorus and Xiphinema transmit polyhedral NEPO viruses such as Arabis mosaic virus, Grapevine fan leaf virus and tomato ring-spot. Trichodorus and Paratrichodorus transmit NETU viruses such as tobacco rattle and pea browning.

2.2.3. 2.3. Animals dispersal: Farm animals can be vectors of disease. They may carry pathogens externally, such as on their body surfaces, especially legs and hooves, or internally through the intestinal tract. While the soil-dwelling fungi that cause rot and wilting are usually introduced from the outside, certain smut fungi that cause disease in crops are transmitted through the intestinal tract.

2.2.3.2.4. Birds dispersal: Birds play a very minor role in disease transmission, but they do occur in seed dispersal from higher flowering parasites. Loranthus sp. parasitic on certain trees such as mangoes.

2.2.3.2.5. Equipment dispersal: Agricultural equipment used in cultivation often transmits plant pathogens from one location to another. Pathogens in this case are usually carried in the form of plant disease residues present in the soil. Similar tools used to perform tasks such as cutting, pruning, sprouting, grafting and thinning. It also helps in transmitting certain diseases from plant to plant. Some viral diseases are spread through budding and grafting operations.

2.2.3.8. Human dispersal: Humans are often involved in the transmission of plant diseases in two ways.

- Workers who handle seedlings, other planting material or fruit may come into personal contact with plant pathogens such as fungi and bacteria. When handling diseased material and unwittingly transferring pathogens to healthy seedlings or plant parts through contaminated hands. This is a kind of "continuous" transmission mode.
- The alternative, or "discontinuous" transmission pathway for which humans are solely responsible, is between geographically distant areas, often separated by physical barriers such as oceans, mountains, and deserts. This is the most efficient and equally dangerous phenomenon of plant disease transmission. Such long-distance transmission of the disease to previously unaffected areas and countries is usually via transportation of infected seeds, seedlings, or timber. So this is a kind of direct transmission through the propagating substance.

7

Role of Environment and Host Nutrition on Disease Development

Disease development depends on three factors: host, pathogen, and environment.

- Host must be susceptible.
- The pathogen must be virulent to cause disease.
- The environment must be conducive to disease development.

Role of environment on disease development

Environment

- The entire environment includes the entire biosphere with integrated epidemiological processes.
- Easy-to-understand display of the entire environment divided into micro, meso, and macro.
- The microenvironment is the space in which epidemiological processes occur at the cellular and organ level.
- Most of the infectious cycle from deposition to initiation. The leaf microenvironment is called the phyllosphere and contains an air layer up to 1 mm thick that surrounds the leaf.
- The phyllosphere is a three-dimensional space, but the actual leaf surface is a two-dimensional space.
- Roots have a three-dimensional rhizosphere (Hiltner, 1904) and a two-dimensional root surface.
- The mesoenvironment is formed by culture. It is formed by plants and simultaneously influences epidemiological processes in plants and cultures.
- The macroenvironment is the layer of air from the surface of plants to the troposphere.

- Several epidemiological processes of great importance occur in the macroenvironment.
- Several environmental factors contribute to disease development by altering host metabolism and/or pathogen virulence.
- This chapter describes various environmental factors that contribute to the development of disease.

A. **Atmospheric environment**

1. Temperature
2. Moisture
3. Wind
4. Light

B. **Soil environment**

1. Moisture
2. Soil temperature
3. Soil pH

A. **Atmospheric environment**

1. Temperature

- Temperature effects
    - Incubation period: the time from infection to the first appearance of symptoms of the disease.
    - Generation time: Time from infection to sporulation.
    - Infectious period: The period during which the pathogen continues to multiply.
- Warmer temperatures accelerate disease cycles, resulting in faster outbreaks of epidemics.
- The epidemic usually progresses slowly in cool environments. Therefore, disease incidence and severity may not reach the thresholds required to cause significant crop loss.

1.1. Effect of temperature on pathogens

- Temperature can encourage the growth of pathogens.
- It leads to the incidence of serious diseases.

- The optimum temperature for the growth of *Xanthomonas campestris* pv. *oryzae*, the pathogen of rice wilt, is 25-30°C.
- Temperatures above 25°C are more likely to cause disease.
- No symptoms at temperatures below 20°C.
- *Puccinia striformis*, the causative agent of wheat rust, does not tolerate high temperatures. Both spores and mycelium grow best around 11°C.
- Few diseases occur in seasons with temperatures above 25°C.

1.2 Predisposing effect of temperature on the host

- Blast explosion is serious due to low night time temperatures.
- Rice produces more L-glutamine when the temperature is 20°C.
- Glutamine stimulates the germination of *Pyricularia oryzae* spores, the causative agent of the blast.
- The nitrogen level rises at lower temperatures, which reduces the production of phenol.
- Phenol is toxic to fungi and low phenol content promotes disease development.
- The optimum temperature for growth of the tobacco root rot pathogen *Thielaviopsis basicola* in culture is 28°C. However, tobacco is most damaged at temperatures between 17-23°C.
- Increased disease incidence is due to poor host growth at low temperatures. A weakened host is severely affected by the pathogen.

1.3. Examples

- Root rot caused by *Macrophomina phaseolina* is severe even at high temperatures (30-35°C).
- Powdery mildew occurs at high temperatures.
- Bean powdery mildew (*Erysiphe cichoracearum*) and green powdery mildew (*Erysiphe cichoracearum*) are very prominent in summer.
- Tobacco mosaic virus severely affects beans at high temperatures.
- Rice blast is a low-temperature disease becomes more severe when nighttime temperatures fall below 20°C.

- Cotton verticillium wilting is severe at low temperatures.
- Wheat smut is severe at temperatures around 19-20°C Disease does not occur at high temperatures (29-30°C).

2. Moisture

- Humidity is the most important environmental factor affecting the development of fungal, bacterial and nematode diseases.
- The term "moisture" includes precipitation, relative humidity, dew, and leaf moisture.
- The impact of rain spray and running water on pathogen spread is also important.
- Leaf moisture is a more accurate indicator of disease than precipitation or thaw.
- In many cases, the combination of leaf wetness and ambient temperature is critical to the spread of host-infecting pathogens.
- Moisture has a significant impact on the spread of pathogens.
- The effect of free water or raindrops facilitates the release and spread of many fungi and almost all bacteria.
- This is a very useful adaptation for pathogens, as breeding conditions are likely also favorable for germination and infection.
- The impact of raindrops releases many dried spores.

2.1 Humidity

- *Peronosclerospora sacchari*, the causative agent of sugarcane downy mildew, produces more conidia when the relative humidity increases from 86% to 95%.
- Sorghum downy mildew (*Peronosclerospora sorghi*) sporulation is maximized at 100% relative humidity. Conidia will not form below 80% relative humidity.
- Humidity also alters host physiology.
- Ragi grown in a very humid environment is low in sugar, and low sugar levels are more susceptible to *Helminthsporium nodurosum* leaf blight.

2.2. Dew

- Dew supports sporulation of many fungal pathogens.
- *Peronospora philippiensis*, the causative agent of sorghum downy mildew, produces conidia when the leaves are moist for at least 4-5 hours. Dew must be present for sporulation to occur.
- The freezing period is very important for the development of rice blast. Dew promotes germination of Pyricularia conidia. A 6-8 hour freezing period favors the disease.

2.3. Rain

- Spore dispersal is caused by rain.
- Downy mildew (*Sclerospora graminicola*) spreads sporangia up to 340 meters in the wet season. However, during the dry season the spread is only up to 80 meters.
- Frequent drizzle is predisposing to bajra ergot (*Claviceps fusiformis*).
- Rice wilt (*Xanthomonas campestris pv. oryzae*) becomes severe after the onset of heavy rain. Rain spreads bacteria and causes epidemics.

3. Wind

- After strong winds, rice diseases become more severe.
- Strong winds can seriously damage to leaf.
- Wound injury facilitates invasion of host leaves by bacteria (*X. campestris pv. oryzae*).

4. Light

- Light is known to sporulate fungal pathogens.
- Longer light periods promote sporangia formation in *Sclerospora graminicola*, which causes bajra downy mildew.
- However, sporangia release occurs in the dark.
- Tobacco necrosis virus infection in tobacco is severe at low light levels.
- Under high light intensity the disease is negligible and few lesions appear. Shading increases the appearance of brow spots (*Helminhosporium oryzae*).
- Shade has less sugar and less phenol content. Less phenols lead to more diseases.

B Soil environment

1. Soll temperature

- Cotton is attacked by two wilt pathogens.
- *Verticillium albo-atrum* causes severe wilt at low soil temperatures (about 20°C).
- *Fusarium oxysporum* f.sp. *vasinfectum* causes severe wilting when soil temperature rises to 32°C.

2. Moisture

- Detect outbreaks of soil borne diseases.
- Soil moisture depends on the amount of water present in the soil.
- Water is soil in terms of potential energy called water potential.
- Water potential is defined as the working capacity relative to the working capacity of pure free water.
- The lower the water potential, the greater the water stress.
- Soils have two types of water potential.
- Matrix water protection and seepage water potential.
- The matrix water potential depends on the water content of the soil, while the permeable water potential depends on the salinity of the soil water. Soil water potential is the sum of matrix potential and seepage potential.

- **Example**
  - *Fusarium solani* grows well between -10 and -30 bar and is only prevented when the water potential approaches or drops below -100 bar.
  - Wilt caused by *Fusarium solani* blight is severe in dry soils and rarely or never occurs in moist soils.
  - Potato scab due to *Streptomyces scabies* is severe during the dry season. Diseases are negligible in moist soil.
  - *Phytophthora cinnamomi* grows optimally below -5 bar and does not grow at all below -50 bar water potential. Ø Disease control by pathogens is always stronger in moist soils and not in dry soils.

3. Soil pH

- Tomato wilt caused by *Fusarium oxysporum* f. sp. *lycopersici* is also severe at low pH.
- Cotton wilt caused by *Fusarium oxysporum* is severe in acidic pH but almost absent in alkaline soils. In alkaline soils, micronutrients such as zinc and iron required for pathogen growth are not available.
- Pathogens therefore do not multiply well and cause disease.

C. Complexity of weather factors

- In many cases, no single weather factor alone may contribute to disease incidence.
- Several favorable weather factors combine to cause epidemics.
- for example,
- Both rainfall and temperature are considered important factors in late blight outbreaks in potatoes.
- Snowmelt and lower nighttime temperatures favor the development of rice blast, and minimum temperatures and relative humidity favor the development of tikka (late) leaf spot on peanuts.

Role of host nutrition in disease development

- Deficiency of minerals such as nitrogen, phosphorus, potash, manganese, zinc, copper, iron, magnesium and boron disrupts plant metabolism and starves plants.
- Mineral excesses and deficiencies disrupt the nutritional balance necessary for good plant metabolism and interfere with the action of essential elements.
- Mineral deficiencies and excesses make plants less resistant to fungi, bacteria and other diseases.
- The type of symptoms caused by a deficiency of a particular nutrient depends primarily on the function of the particular plant element.
- Nutrient mobility plays an important role in localizing deficiencies.
- For highly mobile elements such as nitrogen and potassium, deficiency symptoms appear mainly on old and mature leaves.
- Deficiencies of slow elements such as calcium, boron and iron are evident in young leaves.

- Deficiency symptoms of moderately mobile elements such as magnesium and sulfur are evenly distributed throughout the plant.

1. Role of various elements in the plants

Macronutrients	Physiological function
Nitrogen	Constituent of proteins, amino acids, enzymes, hormones, chlorophyll
Phosphorus	Constituent of phospholipids, Nucleic acids, ATP
Potassium	Catalyst in nitrate reduction photosynthesis and cambium activity
Calcium	Constituent of middle lamella, activator of enzymes
Magnesium	Part of chlorophyll, Structural integrity of cell components
Sulphur	Component of amino acids
Silicon	Cell wall component
Micronutients	
Boron	Increase mobility of sugars , Essential for cell division, protein synthesis
Zinc	Constituent of enzymes, DNA polymerase
Iron	Constituent of cytochrome, Haemetin enzymes
Copper	Constituent of plastocyanin, Oxidation reduction reactions
Molybdenum	Essential for nitrogen fixation process

- These elements are part of the various fertilizers and organic matter incorporated into the soil.
- Affects plant growth.
- Green plants harbor many microbial parasites/pathogens.
- Therefore, the nutritional status of plants directly affects these microorganisms.

2. Factors affecting the severity of the disease

- Fertilizer amount and type.
- Effects of organic change.
- Mineral concentrations in resistant and susceptible cultivars.
- Correlated conditions affecting mineral availability.

3. Effects of nutrients on plant defense

- The nutritional status of plants influences disease development by promoting disease development or increasing the plant's physiological resistance.
- Plant nutrition influences disease development through host metabolism and growth.

- Increases plant tissue resistance to disease and pathogenic damage through compensation.
- Some potash and phosphorus fertilizers are known to reduce disease severity by inducing host resistance or promoting crop maturity, thereby reducing pathogen virulence .

4. Effect of fertilizers application on plant pathogens and disease development

4.1. Nitrogenous Fertilizers

- Application of higher or lower doses of nitrogen affects disease development in plants.
- Increased application of nitrogen increases many diseases.
  - Rice blast becomes severe in nitrogen applied fields.
  - Split application reduces blast and bacterial blight of rice.
  - Late application of nitrogen increases wheat leaf blotch (*Septoria nodorum*) and powdery mildew (*Erysiphe graminis*).
- The forms of nitrogen fertilizers used (nitrate or ammonium) also influence disease development.
- Some diseases are favoured by nitrate form of nitrogen while others are favoured by ammoniacal form of nitrogen.
- The forms of nitrogen are likely to influence disease/ pathogen through effect on soil pH and microbial activity.

4.1.1. Diseases favoured by nitrate form of nitrogen

- Brown spot (*Helminthosporium orzae*) of rice .
- Sharp eyespot (*Rhizoctonia solani*) of wheat.
- Wilt (*Verticillium albo-atrum)* and scab (*Streptomyces scabies)* in potato.
- Verticillium wilts and root rots due to Pythium .

4.1.2. Diseases favoured by ammonium form of nitrogen

- Wilts (Fusarium spp.) and root rot (*Rhizoctonia* spp.) in rice.
- Leaf spot (*Helminthosporium turcicum)* in maize.
- Sharp eyespot (*Rhizoctonia solani*) in wheat.
- Black scurf (*Rhizoctonia solani*) in potato.

4.2. Phosphorous

- Phosphorus fertilizers are known to reduce disease severity by inducing host resistance and accelerating plant maturity.
- Avoid infection with pathogens that prefer young tissue.
- Phosphorus reduces the severity of all diseases in barley and potato scab and increases the severity of cucumber mosaic virus in spinach and wheat husks.
- Repeated application of phosphate fertilizers delays the onset and severity of *Gaeumannomyces graminis* in barley.
- Septoria glume spot severity was positively correlated with phosphorus rate, but grain weight and grain yield were negatively correlated.
- Potassium use often reduces disease incidence, presumably by increasing plant phenol synthesis.
- Potassium alters clubroot susceptibility in cabbage and scab susceptibility in potatoes.
- Increased levels of potassium mitigated the adverse effects of applied phosphorus.
- Potassium reduces wheat rust, tomato early blight and corn stalk rot, but aggravates rice blast and root nodules.

4.3. Calcium

- Calcium application alleviates bean root rot caused by Rhizoctonia solani, possibly by altering host pectin metabolism.
- Calcium fertilizer application reduces rhizome diseases such as Rhizoctonia, Sclerotia, Botrytis, Fusarium and Erwinia by hardening the plant cell walls and making them more resistant to pathogen invasion.
- Its excessive use increases tobacco decay and common potato scab.

4.4. Magnesium

- Magnesium may reduce susceptibility to pathogens that produced macerating enzymes as long as Ca levels remain sufficient.
- Application of magnesium fertilizers decreases apple scab & late blight of potato.

4.5. Molybdenum

- Application of molybdenum reduces infection of potato tubers by *Phytophthora infestans* and also diminishes incidence of Ascochyta blight on beans and peas.

4.6. Manganese

- Manganese reduces late blight of potato .
- Glycoproteins (lectin) which are associated with resistance of sweet potato to *Ceratocystis fimbriota* (black rot) and potato to *Phytophthora infestans* (late blight) require Mn for activity.
- An adequate supply of Mn is needed to activate the Shikimate pathway, which leads to active defense mechanisms against various pathogens.

4.7. Iron

- Ferric chloride controls rice brown spot.
- Iron fertilizers known to decrease Verticillium wilt of mango and silver leaf of tree.

4.8. Silicon

- Silicon application reduces rice blast (*Pyricularia oryzae*).
- Silicon gives cell walls a greater strength and works as physical barriers to penetration by *Pyricularia grisea* (rice blast) .

5. Effects of sugar on disease development

- Plant diseases he can be divided into two groups based on the sugar content required by the pathogen.
- They are high sugar diseases or low sugar diseases.

5.1. High sugar diseases

- Spraying crops with chemicals such as DDT and maleic hydrazide increased disease incidence.
- Suppress the outflow of sugar from the leaves.
- Termed as 'high sugar diseases'.
- Examples, rusts and powdery mildews.

5.2. Low sugar diseases

- When plants are sprayed with chemicals such as 2.4D that increase sugar efflux.
- Disease increased and termed these diseases as 'low sugar diseases'
- Examples : Spots

8

Host-Pathogen Interaction, Recognition, Concept, Infection and Symptomatology

Host -Pathogen Interaction

- Most often, plants become diseased when attacked by living (biotic) or affected by non-living (abiotic) pathogens.
- In the first case, at least two components *viz.*, host and pathogen must come into contact and interact for plant disease to occur.
- Then, for disease to develop, a third factor, a favorable range of environmental conditions, must also occur.
- The interaction of the three disease factors was often visualized as a triangle called the "Disease Triangle".
- Each side of the triangle represents one of three components.
- The length of each side is proportional to the sum of the disease-promoting properties of each component.
- The more virulent, abundant and active the pathogen, the longer the pathogen side would be and the greater the potential amount of disease range.
- If the three elements of the disease triangle can be quantified, the area of the triangle represents the amount of disease in the plant or plant population.
- If any of the three elements are 0, there can be no disease.
- The disease triangle is also represented as a triangle, with the words of the three components (host plant, pathogen, environment) placed at the vertices of the triangle rather than the sides.

Stages in the development of disease

- In any infectious disease, a series of more or less different events follow one another, leading to the development and perpetuation of disease and pathogens.
- This sequence of events is called the disease cycle.
- A disease cycle involves changes in plants, their symptoms, and pathogens, and continues within and from one growing season to the next.
- Key events in the disease cycle are:
  1. Inoculation
  2. Penetration
  3. Establishment of Infection,
  4. Colonization (Invasion)
  5. Growth and Reproduction of Pathogen.
  6. Dissemination of pathogen
  7. Survival of pathogen

This chapter only discusses inoculation, penetration, establishment of infection, colonization (invasion), and symptomatology. Remaining issues such as pathogen growth and multiplication, pathogen dissemination and survival are discussed in other chapters.

1. Inoculation

- Inoculation is the initial contact of the pathogen with a potentially infective plant part.
- Pathogens that land on or otherwise come into contact with plants are called inoculum.
- The inoculum is part of the pathogen that can cause infection.
- A pathogen inoculum unit is called a propagule.
  - In fungi, the inoculum contains fragments of mycelia, spores, sclerotia (i.e. compact masses of mycelia).

- For bacteria, mollicutes, protozoa, viruses and viroids, the inoculum always consists of whole individuals of mollicutes, protozoa, viruses or viroids.
- For nematodes, the inoculum can be adult nematodes, juvenile nematodes, or eggs.
- In parasitic higher plants, the inoculum can be plant fragments or seeds.

1.1. Types of inoculum

1.1.1. Primary inoculum: The inoculum that survives dormancy in winter or summer and causes primary infection in spring or autumn is called primary inoculum, and the infection it causes is called primary infection.

1.1.2. Secondary inoculum: An inoculation made from a primary infection is called a secondary inoculum and causes a secondary infection.

1.2. Sources of inoculum

- Fungi, bacteria, parasitic higher plants and nematodes produce inoculum on the surface of infected plants, or the inoculum reaches the plant surface when the infected tissue decomposes.
- Viruses, viroids, mollicutes, fastidious bacteria, and protozoa produce inoculum within plants. Such inoculants rarely reach the plant surface in nature. Insects, for example, can be transferred from one plant to another.
- In some fungal and bacterial diseases of perennials, the inoculum is produced in plant branches, stems or roots. In other cases, it may enter the field with seeds, explants, tubers, or other reproductive organs, or come from sources outside the field.
- For many plant diseases in annual crops, the inoculum survives on perennial weeds or alternative hosts, from which they are transmitted to annuals and other plants at any time of the year.

1.3. Landing or arrival of inoculum

- Most pathogen inoculants are passively carried to the host plant by wind, water and insects.
- Airborne inoculants are usually not carried from the air to the surface of the plant by gravity alone and are washed away by rain.

- Certain inoculants in the soil like zoospores and nematodes are attracted to host plants by sugars and amino acids that diffuse from plant roots.
- Vector-borne pathogens are typically delivered to host plants with very high efficiency.

1.4. Prepenetration phenomena

1.4.1. Attachment of pathogen to host

1.4.1.1. Fungi, bacteria and parasitic higher plants

- They first come into contact with the outer surface of the plant organ.
- They must first adhere to the surface of the host before they can invade and colonize the host.
- The reproductive organs of these pathogens have a slimy substance on their surface or tip that consists of a mixture of water-insoluble polysaccharides, glycoproteins, lipids and fibrous substances. It becomes sticky when wet and helps pathogens stick to the plant.
- Powdery mildew does not require free water for infection. Attachment is achieved by the release of the enzyme cutinase from the spores.
- Fungi responsible for vascular wilting, spores do not adhere after hydration and become sticky once they are able to respire and synthesize new proteins.
- The act of attachment often appears to be essential for signaling for subsequent vascular tract expansion and creation of infectious structures.

1.4.1.2. Pathogens such as mollicutes, fastidious bacteria, protozoa, and most viruses

- They are placed directly into cells of plants by their vectors and they are probably immediately surrounded by cytoplasm, cytoplasmic membranes and cell walls.

1.4.2. Spore germination and perception of the host surface

- Spores have mechanisms that prevent germination until they feel such a stimulus or when there are too many spores nearby.
- When spores are stimulated to germinate, they mobilize stored food, such as lipids, polyols and carbohydrates, to form and extend germ tubes toward rapid assembly of cell membranes and cell walls.

- The germ tube is a specialized structure that often grows over a very short distance before differentiating into an appressorium.
- Recognition of plant surface signals by pathogenic fungi appears to be the result of mediated signaling pathways

1.4.2.1. Cyclic adenosine monophosphate (cAMP)

1.4.2.2. Nitrogen-activated protein kinase (MAPK)

1.4.2.1. Cyclic adenosine monophosphate (cAMP)

- cAMP signals are transduced via cAMP-dM-dependent activation of protein kinase A (= PKA) and subsequent phosphorylation of target proteins.
- The main activity of PKA in germ tube development is the recruitment of carbohydrates and lipids to appressorium sites and is therefore essential for the production of functional appressoria.

1.4.2.2. Nitrogen-activated protein kinase (MAPK)

- Signaling pathways for infection-related development are also achieved through nitogen-activated protein kinases (MAPKs) and their upstream regulatory kinases.
- All of these together comprise a functional unit that transmits input signals from the periphery of the cell to the cell nucleus to elicit the expression of appropriate genes.
- A MAP kinase, K1 or P1, regulates appressorium formation in response to a signal from the plant surface but it is also required for invasive growth or viability in its host plant.

1.4.3. Appressorium formation and maturation

- Once the appressoria are formed, they are firmly attached to the plant surface.
- As a result, the appressorium secretes extracellular enzymes, generates physical forces, or both to trigger invasion of the fungus into the cuticle.
- The appressorium must adhere strongly to the surface of the host plant, withstand the invasive physical forces exerted by the fungus, and withstand the chemical action of the enzymes secreted by the fungus.

- The magnitude of the inflation pressure in the appressorium is 40 times the pressure of a typical car tire.
- Appressorium swelling is caused by a large accumulation of glycerol in the appressorium. This high osmotic pressure draws water into the cell, creating a hydrostatic pressure that pushes the thin hyphae (appressorium osmotic cones) outward through the host.
- Recruitment of spore storage products to the developing appressorium and glycerol biosynthesis therein is regulated by the cAMP signaling pathway, but the initial transfer of lipid and glycogen stores to the developing appressorium is also mediated by K1- found to be regulated by MAP.
- Production of invasion hyphae appears to be regulated by the MAP kinase pathway.

1.4.4. Recognition between host and pathogen

- It is believed that when pathogens come into contact with host cells, an initial event occurs that triggers a fairly rapid reaction in any organism that permits or prevents further proliferation of pathogens and the development of disease.
- The nature of the 'initial event' is not known with certainty for host-pathogen combinations.

1.4.4.1. Pathogen components

1.4.4.2. Host components

1.4.4.1. Pathogen components

1.4.4.1.1. Elicitors

- Eliminate pathogen entry prior to or during host entry.
- May have a narrow host range.For example; Elysitin.
- Pathogen cell surface components (β-glucans, chitin, chitosan, etc.) are released by the action of host enzymes (β-glucanases, chitinases, etc.) and some have broad host ranges.
- Some are synthesized and released by pathogens after they enter the host in response to host signals. This includes bacterial harpin proteins

that induce the development of hypersensitivity reactions, certain hydroxylipids, and certain peptides and carbohydrates that induce specific host defense responses, such as the production of phytoalexins.

- Elicitors are considered determinants of pathogen virulence. Its presence causes hypersensitivity (tolerance) responses and initiation of transcription of plant genes encoding various components of defense responses.
- These defenses by the host plant make the pathogen appear non-pathogenic.
- If the initial recognition signal received by the pathogen favors growth and development, disease can be caused. If the signal suppresses pathogen growth and activity, the disease can be terminated.
- However, if the first recognition trigger received by the host elicits a defensive response, pathogen growth and activity may slow or stop and disease may not develop. Disease can develop when the trigger suppresses or bypasses the host's defensive responses.

1.4.4.2. Host components

- Acts as a signal for detection and activation of pathogens.
- Fatty acids in the cuticle of plants activates the production of the cutinase enzyme by pathogens that degrade cutin.
- A host pectingalacturonan molecule that stimulates the production of pectin lyase enzymes by fungi or bacteria.
- Phenolic compounds, such as strigol, that stimulate the activation and germination of some pathogens.
- Isoflavones and other phenols, amino acids, and sugars released from plant wounds activate many genes in certain pathogens, causing infection.
- Host plants can also provide recognition cues for some pathogens through specific surface features such as ridges and furrows, hardness, and release of certain ions such as calcium.

1.4.5. Germination of spores and seeds

- Fungal spores and seeds of parasitic higher plants initially germinate by producing a typical mycelium that infects and grows on the host plant, or a short germ tube that gives rise to a specialized infective structure, the haustorium.

- Some fungal spores germinate by producing other spores. E.g. Sporangia produce zoospores and the teliospores produces basidiospores.
- Most spores can germinate soon after they are matured and released. Dormant spores require varying lengths of dormancy period before germination.
- Spore germination requires proper temperature, high relative humidity, and nutrients that diffuse through the surface of the plant.
- In some cases, spore germination of a particular pathogen is stimulated only by exudates from plants susceptible to that particular pathogen.
- In other cases, spore germination may be inhibited to a greater or lesser degree by substances released by the plant into the surrounding water.
- The number, length, and growth rate of germ tubes, or the number and mobility of motile spores produced by microflora, can be affected by physical conditions such as temperature and humidity, and the type and amount of exudate that plants produce on the surface.
- The direction of movement of motile spores (zoospores) is also regulated by similar factors. Chemical stimuli emanating from stomata, wounds, or root elongation zones; physical stimuli associated with open stomatal structures; and nutrient gradients that exist between wounds and roots.
- Seeds of parasitic higher plants germinate either by producing a radicle that penetrates directly into the host plant or by first producing a small plant that penetrates the host plant through a specialized feeding organ called the haustorium.
- Most of the conditions mentioned above that affect spore germination and germ tube growth direction also apply to seeds. Haustoria is also produced by many fungi.

1.4.6. Hatching of nematode eggs

- Most nematode eggs contain the first juvenile, either pre-oviposition or immediately after oviposition.
- The hatchlings quickly molt to produce second juvenile stage. The hatchling can remain dormant inside the egg for varying periods of time.
- When the eggs finally hatch, 2nd stage juvenile emerge.
- Second stage juvenile find and invade host plants or undergo additional moulting to produce additional juvenile instars and adults.

- Appropriate temperature and humidity conditions are also required for nematode eggs to activate and hatch.
- Upon approaching plant roots, nematodes are attracted to the roots by certain chemical factors associated with root growth, particularly carbon dioxide and some amino acids.
- These factors diffuse through the soil and attract nematodes several inches away from the roots.

2. Penetration

- Pathogens enter plant surfaces directly through cell walls, natural openings or wounds.
- Some fungi use only one of these routes to enter tissues, while others use multiple routes.
- Bacteria usually enter plants through wounds, rarely through natural openings, and never directly through intact cell walls.
- Viruses, viroids, mollicutes, fastidious bacteria and protozoa enter through vector made wounds. Some viruses and viroids can also enter through wounds caused by tools or other means.
- Parasitic higher plants invade the host directly.
- Nematodes enter plants directly and sometimes through natural openings.
- Penetration do not necessarily lead to infections.
- Many organisms actually invade plant cells that are less susceptible to these organisms and do not cause disease. These organisms are unable to progress beyond the invasion stage and die without causing disease.

2.1. Direct penetration through intact plant surfaces

2.1.1. Fungi

- Most common mode of penetration by fungi, oomycetes, and nematodes.
- None of the other pathogens can enter plants directly.
- Non obligate parasites or hemi biotrophs penetrate via fine hyphae produced directly by spores or mycelium.
- Obligate parasites do this through a penetrating peg produced by an appressorium.

- Fine hypha or appressorium is formed at the point of contact between the germ tube or mycelium and the plant surface.
- Microscopic hyphae grow to the surface of the plant and penetrate the cuticle and cell wall by mechanical force and enzymatic softening of the cell wall material.
- Most fungi form appressorium at the end of the germ tube with a flat surface that contacts the surface of the host plant.
- Penetrating peg then grow from the flat surface of the appressorium into the host, penetrating the cuticle and cell wall.
- In most fungal diseases, the fungus penetrates the epidermis and cell walls of the plant, but in some fungal diseases. such as apple scab the fungus penetrates only the cuticle and it remains between the cuticle and the cell wall.

2.1.2. Parasitic higher plants

- Parasitic higher plants also form appressoria and penetration peg at the point of contact between the radicle and the host plant. Invasion is similar to fungal invasion.

2.1.3. Nematodes

- Direct penetration in nematodes is accomplished by repeated back-and-forth thrusts of their stylets.
- Such thrusts finally create a small opening in the cell wall.
- Nematode then inserts its stylet into the cell or the entire nematode enters the cell

2.2. Penetration through wounds

- All bacteria, most fungi, some viruses, and all viroids can enter plants through various types of wounds.
- Wounds used by bacteria and fungi may be fresh or old and consist of damaged or dead tissue.
- Bacteria and fungi that enter through wounds germinate or multiply in wound fluid, rain film, or dew water present in wound .
- The pathogen then invades neighboring plant cells or secretes enzymes and toxins that kill and soften neighboring cells.

- Some viruses and all mollicutes, fastidious vascular bacteria and protozoa enter plants through vector created wounds.
- All four pathogens are transmitted by specific insect species.
- Some viruses are also transmitted by certain nematodes, ticks, and fungi.
- Some viruses and viroids are transmitted through wounds made by human hands and tools.

2.3. Penetration through natural openings

- Many fungi and bacteria enter plants through stomata, hydathodes, nectarthodes, and lenticels .

2.3.1. Stomata

- Stomata are most abundant on the underside of leaves.
- It is about 10-20 x 5-8 mm in size, open during the day and mostly closed at night.
- Bacteria live in the film of water above the stoma and when exposed to water can easily pass through the stoma and enter the pores where they can multiply and cause infection.
- Fungal spores usually germinate on the surface of the plant, with germ tubes growing through the stomata.
- The germ tube forms an appressorium that fits over the stoma, from which thin hyphae usually grow into the stoma.

2.3.2. Hydathodes

- Hydathodes are more or less open pores on leaf margins and leaf tips.
- Although some bacteria use these pores as a means of invading leaves, few fungi appear to enter plants through hydathodes.

2.3.3. Nectarthodes

- Some bacteria enter flowers *via* nectaries, which are nectaries that resemble flukes.

2.3.4. Lenticels

- Lenticells are openings in fruits, stems and tubers filled with loosely connected cells that allow passage of air.

- During the growing season, the lenticels are open and fungi and bacteria enter the tissue through them and grow penetrating mainly between cells.

3. Establishment of infection

- Infection is the process by which pathogens establish contact with susceptible host and procure nutrients from them.
- Following infection, pathogens grow, multiply, or both within the plant tissues and invade and colonize the plant to a lesser or greater extent.
- During infection, some pathogens obtain nutrients from living cells, often without killing the cells or others kill cells and utilize their contents as they invade them.
- During infection, pathogens release enzymes, toxins, and growth regulators etc that may affect the structural integrity of the host cells or their physiological processes.
- In response, the host reacts with a variety of defense mechanisms, which may result in varying degrees of protection of the plant from the pathogen.
- The condition for a successful infection to occur are
    - Plant variety must be susceptible to the particular pathogen and at a susceptible stage.
    - Pathogen must be in a pathogenic stage that can infect immediately without requiring a resting period.
    - Temperature and moisture conditions in the environment of the plant must favor the growth and multiplication of the pathogen.
- When these conditions occur at an optimum, the pathogen can invade the host plant up to the maximum of its potential, even in the presence of plant defenses, and, as a consequence, disease develops.

3.1. Localized Vs Systemic infection

3.1.1. Localized infection

- These infections may remain localized throughout the growing season or spread easily or very slowly.
- Many infections caused by fungi, bacteria, nematodes, viruses and parasitic higher plants are local. They affect a single cell, a few cells, or a small area of the plant.

3.1.2. Systemic Infection

- Pathogens spread from the plant's starting point and invade most or all susceptible cells and tissues throughout the plant.
- Infection spreads more or less rapidly and can affect entire plant organs (flowers, fruits, leaves), large parts of the plant (branches) or the entire plant.
- Infections by fastidious xylem or phloem-dwelling bacteria, mollicutes and protozoa, and natural infections by viruses and viroids are systemic.
- Downy mildew pathogens, smut and rust-causing pathogen also invade the host systemically, with older mycelia degenerating and disappearing, leaving only young mycelia to survive in actively growing plant tissue.
- Vascular wilt fungi and bacteria enter xylem vessels internally, but are usually confined to a few vessels in the roots, stems, or apexes of infected plants.
- Most or all of the plant's xylem vessels are affected only in the final stages of the disease.

3.2. Invasion

- The spread of a pathogen to a host is called invasion.
- Different pathogens, namely fungi, bacteria, nematodes, viruses, viroids, mollicutes, fastidious bacteria, and protozoa, invade their hosts in different ways and to varying degrees.

3.2.1. Fungi

- Most fungi spread to all tissues of infected plant organs by multiplying between cells as intercellular mycelium or directly through cells as intracellular mycelium.
- The fungal pathogen that causes black spots in rose produces a mycelium that grows only in the area between the cuticle and the epidermis (subcuticular colonization).
- The fungal pathogen that causes powdery mildew produces mycelium only on the surface of the plant, but sends the haustoria to the epidermal cells.
- Pathogens that cause vascular wilting invade the xylem of plants.

3.2.2. Bacteria

- Bacteria invade intracellular tissue, but if part of the cell wall dissolves, the bacteria can also multiply inside the cell.
- Bacteria that cause vascular bundle atrophy also invade xylem blood vessels.

3.2.3. Virus and viroid

- Penetrates tissues by moving from cell to cell within the cell.
- Penetrates all types of living plant cells.

3.2.4. Mollicutes and protozoa

- Invasion of the phloem sieve tube and possibly some adjacent phloem parenchyma cells.

3.2.5. Fastidious bacteria

- Some invade the xylem vessels and only the phloem sieve tube.

3.2.6. Nematode

- Most nematodes invade tissues between cells, but some enter intracellularly.
- Many nematodes do not invade cells or tissues at all, but feed by piercing epidermal cells with a stylet.

4. Symptomatology

- Plant pathogens provoke a variety of responses in the host body.
- This creates anomalies that become visible to plants.
- The visible or otherwise detectable manifestation of abnormal plant physiology, development or behavior resulting from a disease is called a symptom.
- Symptoms and signs are usually distinguished.
- Disease symptoms are expressed as the host's response to the pathogen, whereas signs are symptoms of the disease other than those expressed by the host.
- The signs are usually the structure of the pathogen.

- A disease is first recognized by the presence of symptoms and/or signs, and recognition of certain types of symptoms or signs helps in a definitive diagnosis of the disease.

Classification of symptoms

Symptoms fall into three general categories:

1. **Necrotic symptoms**: Symptoms resulting from the cessation of function leading to death.
2. **Hypertrophy/Hyperplasia**: Overdevelopment. Hyperplasia; an abnormal increase in the number of cells in a particular tissue or organ. Hypertrophy; an abnormal increase in size of a plant or part of a plant. It is generally caused by an abnormal increase in cell size.
3. **Hypoplastic;** Under development; abnormally few cells within a particular tissue or organ.

1. Necrotic symptoms

1	Anthracnose	A sunken, dark lesion of necrotic cells in infected part of host plants
2	Blast	Failure to develop fruit.
3	Rotting	Sudden drying and browning of leaves, shoots, or entire branches.
4	Spot	Large, irregular lesions on leaves, shoots, and stems.
5	Canker	A necrotic, often sunken lesion, especially in the bark or bark of trunks and roots of woody plants.
6	Damping-off	A complex of symptoms characterized by rapid death, browning and rotting of germinating seedlings. Shoots may be killed before they emerge, and stems may be attacked in the root collar area, causing shoots to fall, roots to be destroyed, and cotyledons to be attacked. Organizational collapse.
7	Decay	Disintegration of dead tissues.
8	Dieback	Drying, shrinkage, and browning of twigs and branches from the tips inward toward the trunk.
9	Hydrolysis	The water-soaked translucent appearance of leaves, fruits, and green stems due to the extrusion of water from the cells into the intercellular space.
10	Browning	Sudden drying and browning of indeterminate parts of leaves and fruits. Also damage to the bark leading to dehydration and death.
11	Bullet hole	A circular hole in the leaf caused by the necrotic area in the center of the spot
12	Spots	Round, or irregularly discolored dead areas on leaves, fruits, or green stems.

13	Lines or Streaks	They are prominent symptoms consisting of elongated but relatively narrow lesions. These streaks are usually brown in color.
14	Ring spots	Characterized by the appearance of sometimes discolored but mostly necrotic rings on leaves or fruits and stems. Ring spots are a common type of condition caused by viral pathogens.
15	Disintegration	Disintegration and decomposition of dead tissue.
16	Wilting	A flaccid appearance of leaves and shoots resulting from temporary or permanent loss of turgor due to excessive transpiration from leaves and shoots
17	Yellowing	The loss of green color from chlorophyllous tissues, due to the destruction of the chlorophyll and/or degeneration of the chloroplasts, which unmasks yellow pigments.

2. Hypertrophy/Hyperplasia (Overdevelopment) symptoms

1	Anthocyanescence	A reddish or purplish coloration of leaves resulting from abnormal development of anthocyanin pigments.
2	Callus	Tissue overgrowth produced in response to injury or other irritation and which tends to cover a wound, canker, etc.
3	Enation	Enation is a by-product commonly found in the veins or midribs on the underside of leaves. They can be small, large, papillary, or whorled and vary in number.
4	Leaf curl	Abnormal bending or curling of leaves or shoots due to localized overgrowth of one side or specific tissues.
5	Fasciation	Flattening or fusion of organs such as stems, flowers and roots. The cause is unknown, but in some cases the condition is inherited.
6	Witch's broom	A type of overgrowth that develops with many weak shoots or roots unusually bushy.
7	Sarcody	Abnormal tissue bulges out of the sprawling branches and stems.
8	Scabs	Raised, sometimes roughened lesions of more or less circular shape, localized on fruit, tubers, leaves, and stems.
9	Tumor	A localized growth of any part of a plant, usually the roots, trunk or branches of a tree, usually caused by stimulation of plant meristems by pathogens.
10	Virescence	The process by which normally white or pigmented tissue develops chlorophyll and turns green.
11	Wart	Warts are protuberance on the bulbs and stems that generally have a warty or discolored cauliflower-like appearance.

3. Hypoplastic; Under development; abnormally few cells within a particular tissue or organ.

1	Chlorosis	Yellowing of green tissue due to chlorophyll destruction or chlorophyll hypoplasia.
2	Dwarfism	Below average size of a plant or part of its organs.

3	Etiolation	A complex symptom in which the main symptoms are dwarfing of leaves and inflorescences, underdevelopment of stems, and chlorosis.
4	Mosaic	Light green spots on leaves.
5	Rust	A rough or corky surface forms in places where it would not normally occur.
6	Suppression	Complete prevention of organ development.
7	Shrinkage of leaves	Infected leaves generally shrink due to reduced leaf tissue growth, but veins and midribs remain normally developed.
8	Leaf curling	These symptoms represent irregular and extensive wrinkling and furrowing of the leaves due to reduced vein growth compared to lamellar tissue growth, resulting in sunken veins and lamellar tissue bulges producing curly hairs that guide the leaves.

5. Signs

Signs fall into three general categories:

5.1.Vegetative structures

5.2.Reproductive structures

5.1. Vegetative structures

Mycelium, haustorium, pathogen cells, rhizomorph, sclerotia, etc are structures generally observed.

5.2. Reproductive structures

Apothecia acervuli, asci, basidium, cleistothecium, conidiophores, mildews, perithecia, pycnidia, sporangium, spores, sporodochium etc are the structures commonly observed.

Some major symptoms based on presence of reproductive structures are :

a) **Bunting:** A fungal disease in which the grain contents are replaced by odorous smut spores.

b) **Mildew**: Mildew is a plant disease in which the pathogen is found as a growth on the surface of the host. They appear as white, gray, tan, or purple spots of various sizes on leaves, herbaceous stems, or fruits. In downy mildew, the surface growth is a tangled, cottony or downy layer, whereas in powdery mildew, the surface growth of the fungus is spore-formed in huge numbers and becomes dusty or powdery. Small black fruiting bodies can also occur in powdery clumps.

c) **Rust:** Rust appears as pustules of relatively small spores that usually pass through the host's epidermis. The pustules are dusty or compact and red, brown, yellow, or black in color.

d) **Smut:** The term smut means sooty or carbonaceous powder. Affected parts of the plant show black or purplish-black dusty powder. These symptoms usually appear on the flower organs, especially the ovary, but also on stems, leaves and roots.

e) **Sooty mold**: A coating of soot on leaves and fruits formed by black hyphae of fungi living in honeydew secreted by insects.

9

Disease Development; The Role of Enzymes, Toxins and Growth Regulators

Enzymes, toxins, growth regulators, and polysaccharides are much more common and perhaps more important in the development of plant diseases. The pathogen produce these substances when grown on certain substrates (inducible). Let's talk carefully one by one

1. Enzymes in plant diseases.
2. Toxins in plant diseases.
3. Growth regulator in plant diseases.
4. Polysaccharides in plant diseases.

1. Enzymes in plant diseases

- Enzymes are generally large protein molecules.
- Catalyzes organic reactions in living cells and in solution.
- Each enzyme, which is a protein, is encoded by a specific gene.
- Some enzymes are always intracellular (constitutive).
- Many are produced only when required (induced) by cells in response to internal or external gene activators.
- Each type of enzyme often exists in multiple forms known as isoenzymes.
- Isozymes have the same function, but may differ from each other in some properties, requirements, and mechanisms of action.
- Most of the chemical reactions that occur in cells are enzymatic, so there are almost as many types of enzymes as there are chemical reactions.

1.1. Enzymatic degradation of cell wall substances

- The aerial surface of plants is mainly composed of cuticle and cellulose, whereas the root cell wall surface is composed only of cellulose.
- Epidermal cell walls may also contain suberin and lignin.
- Degradation of each of these substances is brought about by the action of one or more enzymes secreted by the pathogen.

1.1.1 Cuticle wax

- Plant waxes are found as a continuous layer outside or inside the cuticle of many above-ground parts of plants.
- Pathogen. like *Puccinia hordei* produces an enzyme that can break down wax.

1.1.2.Cutin

- Cutin is the main component of the cuticle.
- Many fungi and some bacteria produce cutinases and/or non-specific esterases an enzyme that degrades cutin.
- *Botrytis cinerea,* the causative agent of many plant diseases, produces cutinase and lipase, both of which degrade cutin.

1.1.3. Pectin substance

- Pectin substances form the main component of the middle lamellae.
- Some enzymes break down pectic substances and are known as pectinase or pectolysis enzymes.
- Bacterial wilting of solanaceous plants caused by *Ralstonia solanacearum*, pectin-degrading enzymes are both essential for disease development due to accelerated colonization and increased bacterial attack.
- Anthracnose, caused by the fungus Colletotrichum, produces pectin lyase, a key virulence factor in disease development.
- Pectinolytic enzymes are produced and play a role in the ability of nematodes such as root-knot nematodes, *Meloidogyne javanica*, to penetrate root tissue.
- Pectin enzymes are produced by spore germination and appear to be involved in host invasion along with other virulence enzymes (cutinases and cellulases).

1.1.4. Cellulose

- Cellulolytic enzymes (cellulases) produced by some plant pathogens, bacteria, nematodes, and parasitic higher plants.

1.1.5. Functions of cellulase enzymes

- Softening and dissolution of cell wall material in living plant tissues.
- Facilitation of pathogen entry and spread into the host.
- In addition, it is indirectly involved in disease development by releasing soluble sugars from cellulose chains that feed on pathogens, and in vascular disease it releases large molecules of cellulose into the transpiration stream, interfering with the normal movement of water.
- Bacterial wilt of tomato was caused by the bacterium Ralstonia (Pseudomonas) solanacearum, and the latter required a production of endocellulase for it to become pathogenic and cause disease.

1.1.6. Pectin substances

- Pectin substances form the main component of the middle lamellae.
- Some enzymes break down pectic substances and are known as pectinasc or pectolysis enzymes.
- Pectin methylesterase removes small branches from pectin chains.
- A pectinase called polygalacturonase breaks down pectin chains by adding water molecules to break (hydrolyze) the bond between two galacturonan molecules.
- Pectinases, called pectin lyases, break chains by removing a water molecule from the bond, thereby breaking the chain and releasing a product with an unsaturated double bond.
- Polygalacturonases and pectin lyases include cleaving pectin chains at random points (endopectinase) to release shorter chains or cleaving only the terminal bonds of chains (exopectinase) to produce single There are types that release galacturonan units.
- A pectolytic enzyme that has been shown to be involved in the development of many fungal and bacterial diseases, especially those characterized by soft tissue decay.

1.1.7. Cellulose

- Cellulose is a polysaccharide.
- Cellulolytic enzymes (cellulases) produced by some plant pathogens, bacteria, nematodes, and parasitic higher plants.
- **Role of cellulolytic enzymes**
- Softening and dissolution of cell wall material in living plant tissues.
- Facilitation of pathogen entry and spread into the host.
- Disintegration and dissolution of cell structures.
- It supports pathogens in the development of disease.
- In tomato wilt, bacterial production of endocellulase was required for the latter to become pathogenic and cause disease.

1.1.8. Hemicellulose (Crosslinked glycans)

- A complex mixture of polysaccharide polymers.
- Hemicellulose is a major component of primary cell walls.
- Several hemicellulases appear to be produced by many plant pathogens.
- Certain enzymes called xylanases, galactanases, glucanases, arabinases and mannose produced by pathogens in response to monomers released from the polymers they act on.
- Non-enzymatic degradation of hemicellulose by reactive oxygen, hydroxyl, and other radicals generated by fungal attack also occurs.
- Fungal pathogens produce these enzymes and oxidants, but it is not yet clear how they contribute to cell wall degradation and the pathogen's ability to cause disease.

1.1.9. Lignin

- Lignin is an amorphous three-dimensional polymer.
- The most common basic structural unit of lignin is the phenylpropanoid.
- Most of the world's lignin is degraded and utilized by a group of basidiomycetes called white rot fungi.
- White rot fungi secrete one or more enzymes (ligninases) that make lignin available.

- Some ascomycetes and imperfect fungi, and even some bacteria appear to produce small amounts of lignin-degrading enzymes, causing soft rot cavities in established wood.

1.1.10. Suberin

- Suberin is found in certain tissues of various underground organs such as roots, tubers, stolons, and epidermal layers such as cork and bark tissue.
- Suberin is also formed in response to injury and pathogen defense of specific organs and cell types.
- Typical suberization occurs, for example, in potato tuber cuts, where browning and crusting develop in the form of multi-layered areas with alternating polyaliphatic and polyaromatic layers. These layers are impermeable, strengthen the cell wall and limit water loss through the wound.`
- Plants appear to produce enzymes that synthesize suberin, but it is not known if or how pathogens degrade suberin during infection.

1.2. Enzymatic degradation of substances contained in plant cells

- Most types of pathogens live all or part of their life in association with or within living protoplasts.
- These pathogens apparently obtain their nutrients from protoplasts.
- Some nutrients like sugars and amino acids are molecules small enough to be taken up directly by pathogens.
- However, some of the other plant cell components such as starches, proteins and fats are only available after being broken down by enzymes secreted by the pathogen.

1.2.1 Starch

- Starch is the most important reserve polysaccharide in plant cells.
- Starch is a glucose polymer and exists in two forms, amylose and amylopectin.
- Most pathogens use starch and other reserve polysaccharides for their metabolic activity.
- Starch is broken down by the action of an enzyme called amylase.

- The end product of starch breakdown is glucose, which is used directly by pathogens.

1.2.2. Protein

- Plant cells contain a variety of proteins that play a variety of roles as catalysts (enzymes) and structural materials (membrane and cell wall) for cellular reactions.
- All pathogens appear to be able to degrade many types of protein molecules.
- Plant pathogenic enzymes involved in proteolysis are proteases or proteinases, sometimes peptidases.

1.2.3. Lipids

- Plant cells contain various types of lipids (oils).
- The most important are phospholipids and glycolipids.
- Both, along with proteins, are major components of all plant cell membranes.
- Several fungi, bacteria and nematodes are known to be able to break down lipids.
- Lipolytic enzymes called lipases, phospholipases, etc. hydrolyze the release of fatty acids from lipid molecules.
- Fatty acids are probably used directly by pathogens.

Table. Cell wall and membrane degrading enzymes produced by certain plant pathogens

Enzymes	Substrate	Pathogen
Cutinases	Cutin	• *Fusarium solani* • *Colletotrichum gloeosporioides*
Cellulases	Cellulose	• *Erwinia carotovora* • *Ralstonia solanacearum* • *Aschochyta pisi* • *Rhizoctonia solani*
Hemicellulases	Hemicellulose	• *Sclerotium rolfsii* • *Erwinia carotovora* • *Penicillium expansum*
Proteinases	Protein	• *Rhizoctonia solani* • *Sclerotium rolfsii*
Ligninases	Lignin	• *Botrytis cinerea* • *Heterobasidium annosus*
Esterases	Suberin	• *Fusarium solani* f.sp.*pisi*

2. Microbial toxins in plant diseases

2.1. Definitions

A "toxin" can be defined as a low molecular weight non-enzymatic microbial product that is toxic to higher plants.

2.2. General properties of toxins

- Toxins, are highly toxic substances and are effective at very low concentrations.
- Toxins act directly on the protoplasts of the living host, severely damaging or killing plant cells.
- Many toxins exist in multiple forms with varying potencies.
- Fungi and bacteria can produce toxins both in infected plants and in the culture medium.
- Toxins damage host cells by impairing cell membrane permeability or by inactivating or inhibiting enzymes, thereby preventing proper enzymatic reactions.
- Certain toxins act as antimetabolites, causing a deficiency of essential growth factors.
- Toxins are distinguished from other microbial products such as 'mycotoxins' and 'antibiotics' which are toxic to animals and microorganisms.

2.3. Toxin classification

Toxins are classified as:

2.3.1. Phytotoxins

2.3.2. Vivotoxins

2.3.3. Pathotoxins

2.3.1. Phytotoxins

- Toxins produced by pathogens that are toxic to plants but are not believed to be of major importance during pathogenesis are called phytotoxins.
- Phytotoxins refers to nonspecific toxins.

2.3.2. Vivotoxins

- Toxins that are produced endogenously (in infected tissues) and are involved in the development of disease, but not as the causative agent, are called vivotoxins.

2.3.3. Pathotoxins

- Pathotoxins are toxins that are major determinants of disease and virulence.
- Pathotoxins induce all typical symptoms at reasonable levels and are associated with virulence.
- Host-specific toxins can be considered pathotoxins.

2.4. Classification of toxins based on host specificity

2.4.1 Non-host-specific or non-host-selective toxins

2.4.2. Pathotoxins include toxins that are host-specific.

2.4.1. Non-host specific or Non-host selective toxins

1. A toxin that affects a variety of host plants.
2. Toxicity produced by phytopathogenic microorganisms known to cause disease syndromes in whole or in part not only on the host plant, but also on other plant species not normally affected by the pathogen in nature.
3. Toxins called non-host specific or non-host selective toxins.
4. These toxins increase the severity of diseases caused by pathogens.
5. They influence the virulence of pathogens, but are not essential for pathogens to cause disease.
6. It does not determine the pathogenicity of pathogens.
7. Examples: tabtoxin, tentoxin, phaseolotoxin, cercosporine

2.4.2. Host-specific or host-selective toxins

- A host-specific or host-selective toxin is a substance produced by a pathogenic microorganism that, at physiological concentrations, is toxic only to the pathogen's host and has little or no toxicity to non-susceptible plants.
- Most host-specific toxins must be present for the producing organism to cause disease.

- Host-specific toxins known to be produced only by certain fungi (Cochliobolus, Alternaria, Periconia, Phyllosticta, Corynespora, and Hypoxylon).
- Contains pathogenic toxins
- Examples: T toxin, Victorin or HV toxin, HC toxin.

Table Host specific and non host specific toxins

Host specific toxins			
Toxin	**Pathogen**	**Host**	**Chemical nature**
AK-toxin	*Alternaria kikuchiana*	Pear	Altenin (Furanose ring)
HV- toxin	*Helminthosporium victorae*	Oats	Victoxinine
HC-toxin	*Helminthosporium carbonum*	Corn	Cyclic peptide
AM- toxin	*Alternaria alternata f.sp. mali*	Apple	Alternariolide
AB-toxin	*Alternaria brassicae*	Brassica spp.	Destruxin B
PC-toxin	*Periconia circinata*	Sorghum	Proteinaceous
Host non specific toxins			
Tentoxin	*Alternaria alternata*	Vegetable crops	Cyclic tetrapeptide
Tabtoxin	*Pseudomonas tabaci*	Tobacco	Aminoacid terivative
Alternaric acid	*Alternaria solani*	Potato	Hemiquinone derivative
Cerato-ulmin	*Ceratocystis ulmi*	Dutch elm	Large M. carbohydrate
Pyricularin	*Pyricularia oryzae*	Rice	Nitrogen containing compound
Fusaric acid	*Fusarium spp.*	Corn	5-n-butypicolinic acid

2.5. Pathogenesis and the role of toxins in virulence

- Pathogenicity is a quantitative term that describes the relative ability of a microorganism to cause disease.
- Pathogenicity refers to the ability of an organism to cause disease.
- Changes in host range indicate changes in virulence, and changes in disease severity indicate changes in pathogenicity.
- However, the question arises of when pathogenesis begins and how far the pathogen must spread for successful colonization.
- No toxins required for permeation. Both produced and unproduced toxins enter host tissues.
- Initial colony formation (up to 24 hours) for both isolates is also the same. Only the subsequent invasions differ.

- It is very likely that toxins play an important role only as virulence factors and not as pathogenicity factors.
- In other words, toxins are more important at the necrotic stage than at the biotrophic stage.
- All toxins isolated to date are derived from saprophytic pathogens.
- Toxins were not isolated from obligate parasites such as powdery mildew, downy mildew and rust.

3. Growth regulators in plant diseases

3.1. General features

- Plant growth is regulated by a small group of natural compounds that act as hormones, commonly called growth regulators.
- The major growth regulators are auxins, gibberellins, cytokinins, ethylene and growth inhibitors, which play important regulatory roles in plant life.
- Plant pathogens may produce more of the same growth regulators that plants produce, or inhibitors of the same growth regulators that plants produce.
- They can generate new and different growth regulators or inhibitors of growth regulators.
- Growth regulators act at very low concentrations and even small deviations from normal concentrations can significantly alter plant growth patterns.
- Whatever the mechanism of action involved, pathogens often cause imbalances in the plant's hormonal system, resulting in abnormal growth responses that are incompatible with healthy plant development.
- Pathogens can cause disease by secreting growth regulators into infected plants, as evidenced by a variety of abnormal plant growth responses they provoke, such as inhibition of bud growth.

3.2. Auxin

- The naturally occurring auxin in plants is indole-3-acetic acid (IAA).
- The effects of IAA on plants are:
    - Cell elongation and differentiation.

- Uptake of IAA into the cell membrane.
- Membrane permeability.
- Increased respiration of plant tissue.
- Promotes synthesis of messenger RNA and subsequently protein/ enzyme synthesis.

3.2.1 Elevated auxin (IAA) levels

- Elevated auxin (IAA) levels are found in many plants affected by fungi, bacteria, viruses, mollicutes and nematodes.
- Some pathogens appear to reduce host auxin levels.
- Plant diseases with symptoms caused primarily by auxin overproduction by pathogens.
    - Clubroot of cabbage caused by the pathogen *Plasmodiophora brassicae.*
    - *Exobasidium azaleae* causing azalea leaf and flower gall.
    - Gall produced by peas infected with the bacterium *Rhodococcus fascians*. *Agrobacterium tumefaciens* causing crown gall and the one causing leafy gall of sweet pea and other plants.
    - Root knot of bean plants were infected with Meloidogyne sp.
- Pathogens can not only induce high levels of IAA in their respective hosts, but also produce IAA themselves.
- However, in some diseases, decreased IAA degradation in by inhibition of IAA oxidase is wholly or partially responsible for elevated IAA levels. including corn smut and wheat rust.

Case study

1. Bacterial wilt disease

- More research has been done on several bacterial plant diseases to better understand auxin production and its involvement in plant disease.
- The bacterial wilt of solanaceous plants is caused by *Ralstonia solanacearum*, which causes a 100-fold rise in the IAA level of infected plants compared to that of healthy plants.
- However, the increased plasticity of cell walls brought on by high IAA levels makes the pectin, cellulose, and protein components of the cell

wall more accessible to and may facilitate their degradation by the corresponding enzymes secreted by the pathogen.

- It is unclear how the increased levels of IAA contribute to the development of plant wilt.
- An increase in IAA levels appears to hinder the lignification of tissues, which may lengthen the time that nonlignified tissues are exposed to the pathogen's cell wall-degrading enzymes.
- Auxin impacts cell permeability, which may be the source of the increased transpiration of the infected plants. High IAA levels may also promote higher respiration rates in the diseased tissues.

2. Crown gall disease

- Galls or tumours form on the roots, stems, leaves, ears, tassels, and petioles of host plants in crown gall.
- Disease is caused on by the bacterium *Agrobacterium tumefaciens* that affects more than a hundred different plant species.
- When crown gall bacteria infect new wounds on a susceptible host, crown gall tumours form.
- Cells around a wound immediately begin to create different phenolic chemicals and get triggered to divide.
- Agrobacterium bacteria attach to cell walls rather than invading them, and when they come into contact with phenolic substances like acetosyringone and other signals, they get activated and start processing the DNA in their Ti plasmid, which stands for tumor-inducing plasmid.
- The plant cells are somehow prepared and rendered receptive to a piece of bacterial plasmid DNA (called T-DNA, for tumour DNA) during the intensive cell division during the second and third days following injury.
- A single strand of T-DNA is excised from the Ti plasmid by proteins encoded by genes in the T-DNA virulence (Vir) region, and is then transferred as a TDNA-protein complex into the plant cell nucleus.
- When part of the T-DNA's genes are activated, they contribute to the manufacture of auxins and cytokinins, which turn normal plant cells into tumour cells.
- The T-DNA is subsequently integrated into the nuclear plant DNA (chromosomes) in this way.

- The host plant can no longer regulate the organisation, pace of development, or rate of division of tumour cells as they go on to grow and divide independently of the bacteria.
- Genes that code for opianes are also found in the integrated T-DNA.
- Opines produced by transformed plant cells, which are solely accessible to intercellular life, cultivating crown gall bacteria for food.
- High IAA and cytokinin levels alone cannot transform healthy cells into tumour cells, even though the increased levels of IAA and cytokinins in tumour cells are sufficient to cause the autonomous enlargement and division of these cells once they have been transformed into tumour cells.
- It is unknown whether additional factors or substances contribute to the conversion of normal cells into tumour cells.

3. Knot disease

- Another hyperplastic disease produced by the bacterium *Pseudomonas savastanoi* is the knot disease of olive, oleander, and privet.
- In this disease, the pathogen creates IAA, which causes affected plants to grow galls. The severity of a strain's symptoms increases with the amount of IAA it generates.
- Gall development is not induced by strains that do not generate IAA.
- However, some IAA synthesis is also carried out by a gene in the bacterium's chromosome.
- The bacterial genes for IAA biosynthesis are on a plasmid carried in the bacterium.

4. Leafy gall disease

- The bacteria *Rhodococcus fascians* causes the leafy gall disease, which affects many plants.
- Leafy galls with centres of overgrown shoots and stunted shoot development are formed.
- The bacteria is primarily found on the tissues' outer surfaces, although it can also develop inside in the plant.
- The bacteria in cultured and infected tissues produces auxin, cytokinins, and other hormones.

- In tissues that have previously undergone differentiation, signals from bacteria that are involved in the emergence of symptoms start fresh cell divisions and shoot meristem creation.
- The bacterial signals come from genes on a linear plasmid and have far more sophisticated and distinct functions than only cytokinins.

3.2.2 Gibberellin

- Gibberellin was first isolated from *Gibberella fujikuroi*, the causative agent of bakanae disease
- Foolish rice seedling disease, in which rice seedlings infected with the fungus *Gibberella fujikuroi* grow rapidly and are much taller than healthy plants, is likely the result of gibberellins secreted by the pathogen.
- The most famous gibberellin is gibberellic acid.
- Compounds such as vitamin E and helmintsporol also have gibberellin-like activity.
- Gibberellin has a growth promoting effect.
  - Accelerates the growth of dwarf varieties to normal size.
  - Promote flowering.
  - Stem and root elongation.
  - Fruit growth.
  - Induces IAA formation.
- Auxins and gibberellins also act synergistically.
- Gibberellins appear to activate genes that were previously 'off'.
- Treatment with gibberellin corrected the growth retardation in tobacco and maize plants that had been badly infected with the Etch virus and maize stunting spiroplasma, respectively.
- Gibberellin sprays were also successful in reversing axillary bud suppression, which was brought on by the prunus dwarf virus (PDV) in cherry and the leaf curl virus in tobacco.
- The same therapy also led to an increase in fruit output in cherries with PDV infection.
- The symptoms return on the plants after gibberellin administrations are ceased in the majority of these treatments, even if the pathogen itself does not appear to be impacted.

- However, given that the growth of even healthy plants is similarly boosted following gibberellin treatments. It is unknown if the pathogen-induced stunting of plants is truly caused by a lower gibberellin concentration in the diseased plant.

3.2.3. Cytokinins

- Cytokinins are found at very low concentrations in green plants, seeds and sap.
- Cytokinin is a potent growth factor required for cell growth and differentiation.
- It suppresses the degradation of proteins and nucleic acids, thus suppressing aging.
- The first identified compound with cytokinin activity was kinetin, which was isolated from herring sperm DNA and does not occur naturally in plants.
- Cytokinin activity is increased in galls, crown galls, black galls, rust galls, and rust-infected bean leaves.
- Cytokinin activity is reduced in sap and tissue extracts from cotton plants infected with verticillium wilt and in plants suffering from drought.
- Cytokinins have been implicated in several bacterial galls, including the 'leaf gall disease' of astragalus caused by the bacterium *Rhodococcus* (*Corynebacterium*) *fascians* and witch's broom caused by fungi and mollicutes.

3.2.4. Ethylene

- Produced naturally by plants.
- Ethylene has a variety of effects on plants, including;
    - Chlorosis
    - Cutting leaves
    - Epinasty
    - Stimulation of adventitious roots
    - Fruit ripening
    - Increased cell membrane permeability, a common consequence of infections

- Ethylene is produced by some phytopathogenic fungi and bacteria.
- Ethylene content increases in proportion to (premature) yellowing of banana fruits infected with *Ralstonia solanacearum*, whereas no ethylene is detectable in healthy fruits.
- Ethylene is also associated with leaf birth symptoms of vascular wilt syndrome and premature leaf loss seen in several plant diseases.
- In verticillium wilt in tomatoes, the presence of ethylene at the time of infection suppresses the development of disease, and the presence of ethylene after infection promotes the development of verticillium wilt.

Table : Plant diseases involving altered concentration of growth regulators

Growth Regulators	Role in disease development	
Auxins	**Increased concentration:**	
	Disease	Pathogens
	Crown gall of apple	*Aagrobacterium tumefaciens*
	Stem rust of wheat	*Puccinina graminis tritici*
	Downey mildew of rucifers	*Puccinia parasitica*
	Wilt of tomato	*Verticillium albo-atrum*
	Wilt of banana	*Fusarium oxysporum* f.sp. *cubense*
	Bacterial wilt of solanaceous crops	*Pseudomonas solanacearum*
	Reduced concentration	
	Potato leaf roll	Potato leaf roll virus
	Curly top of sugarbeet	Sugarbeet curly top virus
	Tobacco mosaic	Tobacco mosaic virus
Gibberellins	**Increased concentration**	
	Bakanae disease of rice	*Gibberella fujikuri*
	Creeping thistle rust	*Puccinia punctiformis*
	Reduced concentration	
	Anther smut of sea campion	*Ustilago violacea*
Cytokinins	**Increased concentrations**	
	Club root of crucifers	*Plasmodiophora brassicae*
	Crown gall of apple	*Agrobacterium tumefaciens*
	White rust of crucifers	*Albugo candida*
	Root knot of tobacco	*Meloidogyne incognita*
	Reduced concentrations	
	Root knot of tomato	*Meloidogyne incognita*
	Verticillium wilt of tomato and cotton	*Verticillium al boratrum*

Growth Regulators	Role in disease development	
Ethylene	**Increased concentration**	
	Wilt of tomato	*Fusarium oxysporum* f.sp. *lycopersici*
	Verticillium wilt of cotton	*Verticillium albo-atrum*
	Wilt of tulip	*Fusarium oxysporum* f. sp. *tulipae*

4. Polysaccharides in plant diseases

4.1. General features

- The role of mucoid polysaccharides in plant disease appears to be particularly important in wilt caused by pathogens that invade the plant's vascular system.
- In vascular wilting, large polysaccharide molecules released by pathogens in the xylem may be sufficient to cause mechanical occlusion of vascular bundles, thereby inducing wilting.
- Exopolysaccharides appear essential for some pathogens to cause normal disease symptoms.
- Exopolysaccharides act by either directly causing symptoms or indirectly promoting disease onset by promoting colonization or promoting pathogen survival.

10

Defense Strategies

Philosophy of defence in plants

- Plants cannot move and must resist or tolerate co-located pathogens.
- Plants have evolved very powerful preformed defense systems in the form of structural and toxic barriers.
- Plants cannot keep intruders out, they can only limit (contain) them.
- Plants can tolerate more nutrient runoff. They often sacrifice a piece of tissue to contain pathogens.
- Poorly developed division of labor requires each cell to perform a function, including defense.
- Plant cells contain antimicrobial substances in their compartments that help the cells self-defense.
- Plant metabolism is affected by environmental conditions and thus defense mechanisms.
- The plant vasculature is inefficient and movement through the apoplast is passive, but the loading of the symplast is highly selective (toxic molecules cannot be transported).
- Each individual plant has its own defense system. Nothing works at population or community level.
- Primitive systems similar to animal immune systems are likely to function. Shared antigenicity in compatible host-pathogen interactions.

Mechanisms of defense used by plants

1. **Pre existing or preformed or passive defense**

- Protection from pathogens is provided by physical and chemical barriers that exist in the host prior to infection.

- The surface layer provides a physical barrier to infection, and toxic chemicals within the surface layer or host cells create an inhospitable environment that prevents pathogen colonization.

2. **Induced or active defense**

- Physical and chemical barriers provide a first line of resistance in the form of protection.
- Active dynamic mechanisms are set in motion when defenses fail and pathogens manage to invade plants. So-called defense

Two types

1. **Pre existing or passive defense** (Defense present on or inside the plant since beginning)

    1.1 Pre existing structural defense

    1.2 Pre existing biochemical defense

2. **Post infection or active defense** (Defense in response to attack by the pathogen)

    2.1 Post infection structural defense

    2.2 Post Infection or Induced biochemical defense

1. Pre existing or Passive defenses

1.1. Pre existing structural defenses

1.2. Pre existing biochemical defense

1.1 Preexisting structural defenses

- A plant's first line of defense against pathogens is its surface.
- In order for pathogens to infect, they must attach and enter.
- Several structural defense mechanisms already exist in plants before pathogens come into contact with them.

1.1.1. Wax and cuticle covering epidermal cells.

1.1.2. Structure of the epidermal cell wall.

1.1.3. Stomata and lenticels.

1.1.4. Presence of thick-walled tissue that impedes the spread of pathogens to plants.

1.1.1. Wax and cuticle that cover the epidermal cells

- Waxes on leaves and fruits form a water-repellent surface.
- This prevents the formation of a film of water in which pathogens can settle and grow (bacteria) or germinate (fungi).
- Thick matting hairs on the surface of plants can provide a similar water repellent effect and reduce infection.
- A thick cuticle may increase resistance to infection by diseases that enter the host only through direct entry of pathogens.

1.1.2. Structure of the epidermal cell walls

- Outer wall thickness and toughness of epidermal cells are apparently important factors in plant resistance to specific pathogens.
- Thick and tough walls of epidermal cells make direct penetration of fungal pathogens difficult or impossible.
- Plants with such walls are often resilient.

1.1.3. Size, location, and shapes of stomata and lenticels

- Many pathogens enter plants only through stomata.
- Most pathogens can enter through closed stomata.
- Some, such as wheat stalks rot can only enter if the stomata are open.
- Stomatal structure. Very narrow entrances and widely raised guard cells may also confer resistance to certain bacterial pathogens in some cultivars.

1.1.4. Presence of tissues made of thick-walled cells that hinder the advance of pathogen on the plant

- The cell walls of affected tissues vary in thickness and toughness.
- This may inhibit the progression of pathogens.
- The spread of infections can be inhibited in particular by the existence of bundles or broad regions of dural cells, which are common in the stems of many cereal plants. For example, Stem rust pathogen.
- Many fungi, bacteria, and nematode pathogens that create different "angular" leaf spots are successfully halted by the xylem, bundle sheath, and hard tissue cells of leaf veins.

- Xylem vessels appear to be more directly involved in resistance and susceptibility to vascular disease.
- For example, xylem vessel diameter and proportion of large vessels were strongly correlated with elm susceptibility to dutch elm disease caused by the fungus *Ophiostoma novo-ulni.*

Table. Pre-infectional morphological and structural defense mechanisms against plant pathogens

Sl. no	Defense barrier	Pathogen	Host
1	Waxes and cuticle	*Albugo candida*	Brussels sprout
		Puccinia graminis	Berberries
		Melampsora lini	Linseed
		Colletotrichum cooffeanum	Coffee
2	Structure of natural opening		
	Broad cuticular ridge projection over the stomata	*Xanthomonas campestris pv.citri*	Mandarins citrus
	Mechnical (Sclerenchymatous) tissues	*Entyloma oryzae*	Rice
	Late openining of stomata	*Puccinia graminis tritici*	Wheat
3	Thick and tough outer cell wall (Presence of silicic acid and lignified epidermal cells)	*Pyricularia oryzae*	Rice

1.2. Pre existing biochemical defense

- When biochemical defenses already exist in the plant before the pathogen attacks.
- Plant cells have specific metabolic processes that make them resistant to attack by pathogens.
- This type of plant defense is called 'biochemical defense'.

1.2.1 Release of antimicrobial compounds.

1.2.2 Inhibitors present in plant cells.

1.2.3 Lack of essential elements.

1.2.4 Recognition elements.

1.2.5 Essential nutrients and growth factors.

1.2.6 Common antigens of host plants.

1.3. Release of antimicrobial compounds

- Plants normally excrete organic matter, including amino acids, sugars, organic acids, enzymes, glycosides, etc. from the shoots and roots.

- Some compounds in exudates are inhibitory.
- These inhibitors either act directly on microorganisms or stimulate specific groups to dominate the environment and act as antagonists to pathogens.
- For example,
  1. Certain flax varieties are resistant to *F. oxysporum* infection. This is due to the presence of HCN in root exudates.
  2. The presence of HCN in sorghum and maize roots has also been reported, which has been implicated in the reduction of pigeon pea wilting caused by *Fusarium udum* in plots where sorghum is intercropped with pigeon peas.
  3. Red onion scales (red cultivars) contain protocatechuic acid and catechol, which may bleed into the drip and confer resistance to *Colletotrichum sarcinianus* (Onion spot disease) infestations.
  4. Root exudates promote the development of plant growth-promoting root bacteria (PGPR) that inhibit plant pathogens and induce resistance.

1.2.2. Inhibitor present in plant cells

- Plant cells contain specific pre-existing inhibitors that play a protective role, primarily against pathogens of concern.
- Phenols and quinones are two classes of antimicrobial compounds produced by some plants.
- Lactones, cyanoglucosides, saponins, terpenoids, stilbenes, and tannins are plant-derived compounds associated with pathogen resistance.
- Saponins are a class of plant anticipins that disrupt the membrane integrity of saponin-sensitive parasites released after injury or infection.
- Plant defensins are an additional class of antibodies that prevent pathogens from obtaining nutrients and retard their growth.
- Defensins may be secreted, which can offer an antimicrobial environment for seed germination, and they may accumulate up, which can protect flowers, leaves, and bulbs against insect-borne viruses.
- Additionally, induced and constitutive proteins contribute to plant defence.

1.2.3. Recognition factors

- The first step in the infection process is cell-to-cell communication between pathogen and host.
- Plants of that species or variety should not be infected with pathogens if the surface cells of the plant do not have a specific recognition factor.
- If a pathogen does not recognize a plant as one of its hosts, it may not adhere to the host's surface or produce infectious agents such as enzymes or structures such as appressoria.
- These recognition molecules are various types of oligosaccharides, polysaccharides and glycoproteins.

1.2.4. Essential nutrients and growth factors

- Most obligate parasites and some facultative saprophytes, especially among fungi, are usually host-specific and only grows on certain host varieties.
- Only grows on certain host varieties.
- This happens because host-specific pathogens require specific substances.
- These substances are only present in sufficient amounts in the infected host.
- Thus, the absence of these specific substances renders other varieties unsuitable hosts for such pathogens.
- For example, in some crop seedling diseases caused by *Rhizoctonia solani*, successful infection depends on the formation of an infection cushion, from which foci of infection develop and lead to invasion. Formation of these cushions is induced by certain essential nutrients of the host.
- In resistant plants, deficiency of such nutrients leads to resistance to *Rhizoctonia solani.*
- Mutations can cause a pathogen species to lose its ability to synthesize a particular substance, making the pathogen species non-specific.

1.2.5. Common antigen in host plant

- The presence of common antigens (proteins) in the host and pathogen determines disease development in the host.

- However, if the antigen is not present in the host, but only in the pathogen, the host becomes resistant to that particular pathogen.
- Flax cultivars that share antigens with the pathogen *Melampsora lini* have been shown to be susceptible to rust.
- In contrast, flax cultivars that do not carry the antigen but do have the pathogen present are resistant to the pathogen.
- The same applies to cotton leaf spot caused by Xanthomonas a campestris a malignant bacteria.

Table: Pre-infectional biochemical defense mechanisms against plant pathogens

Sl.No	Defense barrier	Pathogen	Host
1	**Inhibitors released by the plant in the environment**		
	Glucoside	Fusarium spp.	Flax
	Malic acid	*Ascochyta rabiei*	Gram
	Catechol and protocatechuic acid	*Colletotrichum circinans*	Onion
	Cutin acid	*Gloesporium limetticola*	Citrus
2	**Phenolic substances**		
	Polyphenols	*Venturia inaequalis*	Apple
		Pyricularia oryzae	Rice
		Venturia pirina	Pear
3	**Inhibitory substances present in the plant cells**		
	Chlorogenic acid	*Streptomyces scabies*	Potato
	Tuliposide	*Fusarium oxysporum f.sp. tulipae*	Tulip
	Avenacin	*Ophiobolus graminis*	Wheat
	Arbutin	*Erwinia amylovora*	Pear
4	**Absence of nutrients required by the pathogen**		
	Histidine	*Erwinia amylovora*	Potato
	Sugar	*Ceratocystis ulmi*	Elm
		Alternaria solani	Potato
		Cochliobolus sativus	Barley
	Choline	*Venturia inaqualis*	Apple
	Myoinositol	*Rhizoctonia aurecina*	Plum

2. Post infection or active or induced defense

2.1. Post infection or Induced structural defense

- Most plant pathogens enter the host through wounds or natural openings.
- Although the host plant has preformed surface or internal defense structures, pathogens cause different degrees of infection.

- However, even after pathogens invade preformed defense structures, plants typically respond by forming one or more types of structures.
- Its structure more or less successfully protects the plant from further invasion of pathogens.

2.1.1.	Cell wall defense structures	Involve walls of invaded cells.
2.1.2	Cytoplasmic defense reaction	Defense structures formed involve the cytoplasm of the cells under attack.
2.1.3	Histological defense structures	Involve tissues ahead of the pathogen
2.1.4	Necrotic or Hypersensitive defense reaction	Death of the invaded cell may protect the plant from further invasion.

2.1.1 Cell wall defense structures

- Accompanied by morphological changes in the cell wall.
- Changes brought on by pathogens invading cells' cell walls.
- Mainly three types of structures have been observed in plant diseases.
    - The outer layer of the parenchymal cell wall that comes in contact with incompatible pathogens swells and produces substances that surround and trap the pathogens and prevent their growth.
    - Cell walls thicken and produce cellulosic material in response to multiple pathogens. Infused phenolic substances that are cross-linked and further increase resistance to penetration.
    - Callose papillae are deposited inside the cell wall in response to invasion by fungal pathogens. They appear to prevent pathogens from later entering the cell.

2.1.2 Cytoplasmic defense reaction

- The cytoplasm of the plant cell surrounds the hyphal mass and the nucleus of the plant cell is stretched until it splits in two.
- Cytoplasm and nucleus enlargement in some of the affected cells.
- The cytoplasm becomes granular and dense, and various particles and structures appear within it.
- Finally, the pathogen's mycelium is degraded, stopping the invasion.
- For example, weakly pathogenic Armillaria strains and mycorrhizal fungi cause chronic disease or mostly commensal conditions.

2.1.3 Histological defense structures

2.1.3.1.Formation of cork layers

- Infection by plant pathogens often causes plants to grow multiple layers of cork cells beyond the point of infection.
- A layer of cork prevents further penetration of pathogens beyond the initial lesion.
- It also blocks the spread of toxic substances secreted by pathogens.
- The cork layer also stops the flow of nutrients and water from healthy areas to infected areas, depriving pathogens of nutrients.
- Dead tissue containing pathogens is trapped by the cork layer and stays in place forming a necrotic lesion.
- Depending on the host-pathogen combination, the necrotic tissue is pushed outward by the underlying healthy tissue, forming a sloughing scab that completely removes the pathogen from the host.
- Example cork stratification of potato tubers after Rhizoctonia infection.

2.1.3.2. Formation of abscission layers

- Abscission consists of a gap formed between two circular layers of leaf cells surrounding the site of infection.
- Upon infection, the intermediate layer between these two cell layers dissolves throughout the leaf thickness, completely detaching the central region of infection from the rest of the leaf.
- Gradually this area shrinks, dies, sloughs off and carries pathogens.
- A deciduous layer forms on the young vigorous leaves of stone fruit trees after infection with one of several fungi, bacteria or viruses.

2.1.3.3. Formation of tyloses

- Tylose is a protoplast outgrowth of adjacent viable parenchymal cells that protrude from pits into xylem vessels.
- Tylose is formed within the xylem vessels of most plants during invasion and under stress by most xylem-invasive pathogens.
- Tyloses have cellulose walls and, depending on their quantity and size, might totally block the vessel.

- When a pathogen is present in immature roots of some varieties of plants, tyloses grow rapidly and in large quantities ahead of the infection, preventing further disease advancement.
- These plant varieties' continue to be free of and so resistant to this infection.Disease is more likely to affect varieties where few, if any, tyloses occur before the infection.

2.1.3.4. Deposition of gums

- Many types of gums are produced by many plants near the lesion after infection or injury by pathogens.
- They are rapidly deposited in intercellular spaces and cells surrounding the site of infection.
- Forms an impenetrable barrier that completely surrounds pathogens.
- The pathogen is then isolated, starved, and sooner or later dies.
- Gum secretion is most common in stone fruit trees, but occurs in most plants.

Table: Post-infectional morphological and structural defense mechanisms against plant pathogens

Sl.No	Defense barrier	Pathogen	Host
1	Formation of cork layer	*Rhizoctonia solani*	Potato
		Coccomyces prunophorae	Plum
	Formation of tyloses	*Fusarium oxysporum* f.sp *batatas*	Sweet potato
		Verticillium- alboatrum	Tomato
3	Formation of abscission layer	*Xanthomonas arboricola pv. pruni*	Sour cherry
		Clsterosporium carpophilum	Peach
3	Sheathing of hyphae	*Phytophthora infestans*	Potato
4	Gum deposition	*Pyricularia oryzae*	Rice
		Drechslera oryzae	Rice
		Physalopora cydoniae	Apple

2.1.3.4. Defense through the Hypersensitive response

- Hypersensitivity reactions are believed to be biochemical reactions rather than structural defense mechanisms.
- When a pathogen contacts a host cell, the cell nucleus migrates toward the invading pathogen and immediately collapses.
- At the same time brown resinous granules are formed in the cytoplasm. It forms first around the point of pathogen entry and then throughout the cytoplasm.

- A brownish discoloration of the cytoplasm of plant cells persists, and as death begins, the invading hypha begins to degenerate.
- In most cases, hyphae will not grow from such cells, preventing further invasion.
- This type of necrotic defense is particularly prevalent in diseases caused by obligate fungal parasites, viruses, bacteria and nematodes.
- Necrotic tissue isolates the parasite from the organisms it depends on for life, resulting in starvation and death.
- It denotes numerous biochemical cell reactions and antimicrobial concentrations that neutralize pathogens.

2.2. Post infection or Induced biochemical defense

These mechanisms restrict the spread of the pathogen after infection is established and contain the damage to host tissues.

2.2.1. Inactivation of enzymes and toxins

- The role of pathogen enzymes and toxins in pathogenesis is well established.
- Semi-biotrophs and necrotrophs use more of these substances to cause tissue damage to the host compared to biotrophs.
- It is generally known that phenols, tannins, and proteins operate as enzyme inhibitors in defence mechanisms for resistant plants.
- Phenol has no antifungal effect, but neutralizes pathogens by neutralizing their enzymes.
- In unripe grapes, catechol tannins inhibit enzymes produced by *Botrytis cinerea*.
- Released pathogenic toxins from infections are detoxified by the ability of metabolic processes in resistant plant cultivars that develop diseased as a result of those toxins.
- The pathogen Pyricularia oryzae produces picolinic acid and pyricularin toxin in the host, producing blast disease in rice. While susceptible cultivars are attacked by these toxins, resistant cultivars convert 40–60% of picolinic acid to its methyl ester, N-methylpicolinic acid, or pyricuraline.These resistant compounds are non-toxic to rice.

Table. Defense through detoxification of pathogen toxin

Detoxifying compound	Pathogen toxin	Disease	Pathogen
Chlorogenic acid	Piricularin	Blast of rice	*Pyricularia oryzae*
Dehydroascorbic acid	AK toxin	Black spot of pear	*Alternaria kikuchiana*
High concentration of cysteine Fusaric acid		Wilt of cotton	*Fusarium oxysporum f. sp. vasinfectum*
		Wilt of tomato	*Fusarium oxysporum f. sp. lycopersici*

2.2.2. Defense through Pathogenesis-related proteins

- Pathogenesis-related proteins is also called PR proteins.
- PR proteins is a group of structurally diverse plant proteins that are toxic to invading fungal pathogens.
- They are distributed in trace amounts of plants.
- It is produced in much higher concentrations after exposure to pathogens or stress.
- PR proteins are also found in the intracellular and intercellular spaces (cell walls) of plant cells.
- Different plant organs like leaves, seeds, and roots can produce a diverse set of PR proteins.
- PR proteins are either very acidic or very basic, making them highly soluble and highly reactive.
- At least 14 families of PR proteins are recognized.
- Well-known PR proteins are
    - PR1 protein (Antioomycete and antifungal)
    - PR2 (β-1,3-glucanase)
    - PR3 (Chitinase)
    - PR4 protein (Antifungal)
    - PR6 (Proteinase inhibitor), thaumatin-like protein, defensin, thionine, lysozyme, osmotin-like protein, lipoxygenase, cysteine-rich protein, glycine-rich protein, proteinase, chitosanase, peroxidase.
- Numerous genes encoding PR proteins are activated by pathogen attack on healthy plants, trigger treatment, damage, or stress.

- Signaling compounds involved in PR protein induction include salicylate, ethylene, xylanase, polypeptide systemmin, and jasmonic acid.

2.2.2.1. Role of pathogenesis-related proteins

- Antifungal and other antimicrobial activity.
- Inhibit spore release and germination.
- Strengthening of the host cell wall and its outgrowths and papillae.

Table. Families of pathogenesis –related proteins (PRPs)

Sl.No	Protein family	Protein activity	Targeted pathogen sites
1	PRP-1	Unknown	Active against oomycetes
2	PRP-2	B-1,3 glucanase	Cell wall glucan of fungi
3	PRP-3	Endochitinase	Cell wall chitin of fungi
4	PRP-4	Endochitinase	Cell wall chitin of fungi
5	PRP-5	Taumartin-like	Active against oomycetes
6	PRP-6	Proteinase inhibitor	Active on nematodes and insects
7	PRP-7	Endoroteinase	Microbial cell wall dissolution
8	PRP-8	Endochitinase with lysozyme activity	Cell wall chitin of fungi, and mucopeptide wall of bacteria
9	PRP-9	Peroxidase	
10	PRP-10	Ribonuclease activity	Viral RNA
11	PRP-11	Endochitinase	Cell wall chitin of fungi
12	PRP-12	Defensin	Antifungal and antibacterial activity
13	PRP-13	Thionin	Antifungal and antibacterial activity
14	PRP-14	Lipid transfer proteins	Antifungal and antibacterial activity
15	PRP-15	Oxalate-oxidase	Produces H_2O_2 that inhibits microbes and also stimulates host defense
16	PRP-16	Oxalate-oxidase-like with suuperdismutase	Produces H_2O_2 that inhibits microbes and also stimulates host defense

2.2.2.2. Defense through Pathogenesis-related proteins (Examples)

- PR protein component like β-1,3-glucanases and chitinases diffuse toward and affect (degrade) the chitin-supporting structures of the cell walls of some plant pathogens.

- Lysozyme breaks down the glucosamine and muramic acid components of bacterial cell walls.

- Lipoxygenase and lipid peroxidase produce antimicrobial metabolites and secondary signaling molecules such as jasmonate.

- Plant defensins (cysteine-rich peptides) have antibacterial activity and accumulate via the ethylene and jasmonate pathways.
- Plants genetically engineered to express the chitinase gene show good resistance to the soil-borne fungus *Rhizoctonia solani.*
- When tobacco plants were treated with lipopolysaccharides from Gram-negative bacteria's outer wall, they produced a number of PR proteins and systemic responses in the leaves of plants that were inoculated through the roots, including increased production of tobacco defence against Phytophthora nicotianae.

2.2.3. Defense through phytoalexins

- Phytoalexins are antimicrobials produced in significant amounts in plants only upon stimulation or chemical and mechanical injury by various types of phytopathogenic microorganisms.
- They are produced by healthy cells adjacent to local infected and necrotic cells in response to substances diffusing from infected cells.
- Phytoalexins are not produced in compatible biotrophic infections.
- They accumulate around both resistant and susceptible necrotic tissue.
- Resistance occurs when one or more phytoalexins reach concentrations sufficient to limit pathogen development.
- Most known phytoalexins are toxic and inhibit the growth of plant pathogens.
- Some phytoalexins are also toxic to bacteria, nematodes and other organisms.
- Phytoalexins are isoflavonoids and solanaceous terpenoids found in most legumes.
- Phytoalexins include phaseolin found in beans; pisatin in peas; glyceorin in soybeans, alfalfa and clover; lycithin in potatoes; gossypol in cotton; capsidiol in peppers.
- Most phytoalexin elicitors are generally fungal cell wall components such as glucans, chitosans, glycoproteins and polysaccharides.
- Elicitor molecules are released from the fungal cell wall by host plant enzymes.

- Most of these elicitors are nonspecific. They are present in both compatible and non-compatible strains of the pathogen and induce phytoalexin accumulation regardless of plant type.
- Most phytoalexin elicitors are of pathogenic origin. Some elicitors. like galacturonic acid oligomers are either produced by plant cells in response to infection or released from the plant cell wall after partial degradation by pathogen cell wall-degrading enzymes.

Some important phytoalexins

Sl.No	Phytoalexins	Producer plant	Chemical nature
1	Resveratrol	*Vitis vinifera*	Stilbene
2	Trifolirhazin	*Trifolium pratens*	Isoflavonoid
3	Isocoumarin	*Daucus carota*	Isocoumarin
4	Orchinol	*Orchis militaris*	Dihydrophenanthrene
5	Isomeamarone	*Ipomea batata*	Sesquiterpene
6	Rishitin	*Solanum teberosum*	Sesuiterpene
7	Lubimin	*Solanum teberosum*	Sesuiterpene
8	Camelexins	*Aradiopsis thaliana* *Camalenia sativa*	Thiazoyl substituted indole camalexin
9	Brassinins	*Brassica rapa*	Indole ring linked to a dithiocarbamate
10	Pisatin	*Pisum sativum*	Isofalvonoid
11	Maackiain	*Cicer arietinum*	Isofalvonoid
12	Phaseollidin	*Phaseolus vulgaris*	Isofalvonoid

2.2.4 Defense through production of secondary metabolites: Phenolics

- Phenols, the most common compounds found in plants, have aromatic rings with hydroxyl substituents.
- Phenol is toxic to fungi, bacteria and viruses.
- Common phenolic chemicals that are harmful to microorganisms are produced and accumulate more quickly after infection.
- Phenolic compounds produced more frequently in resistant plant cultivars than in susceptible cultivars.
- Examples of such phenolic compounds. Chlorogenic acid, caffeic acid, ferulic acid.
- In date palm roots, cell wall-bound hydroxybenzoic acid and sinapinic acid increased 11- to 12-fold in Fusarium-tolerant cultivars than in susceptible cultivars.

- In peaches, chlorogenic acid is present in fairly high concentrations both in unripe fruits and in berries of cultivars resistant to brown rot caused by the fungus *Monilinia fructicola*.

2.2.4.1. Role of phenol compounds

They inhibit

- Mycelium growth.
- Spore germination.
- Production of cellulose and pectin enzymes.
- Activity of cellulose and pectin enzymes.
- Production of toxins by fungi.

Phenolic substances	**Crop**
Chlorogenic acid	Potato
Catechol and Pyrocatechic acid	Onion
Avenacin	Oats
Hordatine	Barley
Tomatine	Tomato
Tuliposides	Tulip
Catechin and Isoquercitin	Cotton
Umbelliferone and Scopoletin	Sweet potato

11

Altered Plant Metabolism as Affected by Plant Pathogens

Introduction

- Plant pathogens include fungi, bacteria, viruses, viroids, phytoplasma, and nematodes.
- They have evolved different strategies for invading, feeding on, and reproducing inside plants.
- Biotrophic pathogens require living tissue to grow and reproduce.
- Necrotic pathogens kill host tissue at the onset of infection and feed on the dead tissue.
- Viruses generally require living tissue for survival.
- Bacteria and fungi require both biotrophic and necrotrophic strategies.
- Plant pathogens interfere with plant metabolism in one or more ways. These are ;

1. Effects of pathogens on plant growth and reproduction.
2. Effects of pathogens on photosynthesis.
3. Effects of pathogens on water and nutrient migration in host plants.
4. Effects of pathogens on phloem-mediated translocation of organic nutrients.
5. Effects of pathogens on host plant respiration.
6. Effects of pathogens on cell membrane permeability.
7. Effects of pathogens on transcription and translation.

1. Effects of pathogens on plant growth and reproduction

1.1. Effects of pathogens on plant growth

- Destroys part of the root of the plant.
- Clogging of xylem or phloem elements.
- Water movement interventions and of inorganic or organic nutrients.
- Partial destruction of the photosynthetic section of the plant.
- Reduced photosynthetic performance.
- Reduced growth and reduced yield of these plants.
- Reduced plant size and yield, sometimes dying.
- The most common diseases in which pathogens cause apparent overgrowth of host organs and tissues include:
    - Clubroot on cruciferous vegetables caused by *Plasmodiophora brassicae*
    - Wart of potato caused by *Spongospora subterranea.*
    - Peach leaf curl by the fungus *Taphrina* sp.
    - Smut of corn caused by *Ustilago maydis.*
    - Dwarf smut of wheat by Tilletia.
    - Crown gall and hairy apple roots of many hosts caused by *Agrobacterium tumefaciens* and *Agrobacterium rhizogenes.*
    - Olive knot and Oleander knot by *Pseudomonas savastanoi.*
    - Multi-host light gall by *Rhodococcus* sp.

1.2. Effects of pathogens on plant reproduction

Direct effect

- Many pathogens directly affect plant reproduction by directly attacking and killing flowers, fruits or seeds or by interfering with and inhibiting their production.
- Pathogens directly or indirectly interfere with the reproduction of host plants.

Example

- Brown rot of drupes by *Monilinia* sp.
- Bacterial rot of stone fruit trees caused by *Pseudomonas syringae.*
- Fire blight of pears and apples caused by the bacterium *Erwinia amylovora.*
- Ergot of bajra caused by the fungus *Claviceps purpurea.*
- Smut of maize and covered loose smut of various types of cereals caused by Tilletia and Ustilago sp.
- In some diseases caused by viruses, phytoplasma, or phloem-restricted bacteria, no flowers are produced, or the flowers produced are sterile and produce little or no fruit or seeds.

Indirect effects

- Pathogens that attack various plant organs and tissues often weaken and kill those organs and tissues, thereby weakening the plant.
- As a result, such plants will be smaller, with fewer flowers, fewer fruits and fewer seeds.
- The latter may have lower strength and vitality.
- So when you plant, you will get fewer new plants and they can become weaker.

2. Effects of pathogens on photosynthesis

- Pathogen interference with photosynthesis is evidenced by chlorosis, necrotic foci, reduced growth and reduced fruit abundance in many infected plants.
- Photosynthesis is reduced in leaf spots, rot, grain rust and fungal spots, bacterial spots, viral mosaics, yellowing and stunting or defoliation due to reduced photosynthetic surface area of plants.
- The total leaf chlorophyll content is reduced in many fungal and bacterial diseases, but the photosynthetic activity of the remaining chlorophyll appears to be unaffected.
- Photosynthesis is reduced in some fungal and bacterial diseases because the toxins produced by these pathogens, such as tentoxin and tabtoxin, inhibit some of the enzymes directly or indirectly involved in photosynthesis.

- In plants affected by many vascular pathogens, stomata remain partially closed, chlorophyll is reduced, and photosynthesis ceases before the plant eventually dies.
- Most viral, protozoa and nematode diseases also cause varying degrees of chlorosis and stunting, with greatly reduced photosynthesis in infected plants.

3. Effects of pathogens on water and nutrient migration in host plants

Many plant pathogens interfere with the movement of water and mineral nutrients through plants in one or more ways. These are

3.1. Effect on water uptake by roots.

3.2. Effects on water movement through xylem.

3.3. Effects on transpiration.

3.1. Effects on water uptake by roots

- Some plant pathogens impair root integrity and function, making them less water uptake.
- Inhibits root hair formation, alters the permeability of root cells, and inhibits normal water uptake by roots.
- Examples of reducing water uptake by plants
  - Destruction of seedling roots by damping-off caused by Pythium sp.
  - Roots and stems of pepper plants caused by Phytophthora sp.
  - Wheat roots in various stages of destruction by the universal fungus *Gaemanomyces tritici.*
  - Infection of maize canopy and roots by the fungus Fusarium.
  - Numerous bumps on cherry tree roots caused by the bacterium *Agrobacterium tumefaciens.*
  - Knot caused by the nematode Meloidogyne sp. on the roots of cantaloupe plants.

3.2. Effects on water movement through xylem

- Some pathogens impede the movement of water through the stem by growing, for example, in xylem vessels.
- They interfere by their physical presence in the xylem as mycelia, spores

or bacterial cells such as clogging, tylose development and induction of galling in stems and roots.

- Examples of ways to reduce water and mineral nutrient rise
  - Stems of melon plants infected with the fungus Phomopsis sp.
  - Tree canker aof almond caused by the fungus *Ceratocystis fagacearum*.
  - Vascular wilt of tomatoes caused by Fusarium.
  - Discolored vascular tissue in tomato stems infected with the same fungus.
  - Wilted tomatoes infected with the vascular bacterium *Ralstonia solanacearum.*

3.3. Effects on transpiration

- Some pathogens act on leaves and stomata, causing excessive transpiration and disrupting the water balance of the plant.
- This is the result of at least partial destruction of leaf protection by the cuticle, increased leaf cell permeability, and stomatal dysfunction.
- Methods for increasing transpiration of pathogen-infected plants.
  - *Puccinia recondita*, the pathogen of wheat leaf rust, causes numerous lesions (uredia) on wheat leaves, millions of tears on the leaf epidermis, and uncontrolled transpiration. .
  - Uredospores emerging from infected leaf surfaces through the epidermis.
  - Grapeberries infected with the powdery mildew fungus *Uncinula necator* have their mycelium penetrate almost all epidermal cells and form butts there.
  - The apple scab fungus *Venturia inaequalis* grows between the cuticle and the epidermis, causing the cuticle to rupture in various places and allowing transpiration.
  - Tomato leaves with numerous lesions caused by the fungus *Septoria* sp. It is caused by excessive sweating.

4. Interference with movement of organic nutrients through the phloem

- Plant pathogens can interfere with the movement of organic nutrients from leaf cells to the phloem and from the phloem to the cells that use them.

- Obligatory fungal pathogens, such as rust and powdery mildew, accumulate photosynthetic products and mineral nutrients in pathogen-affected areas.
- In these diseases, infected areas are characterized by decreased photosynthesis and increased respiration.
- In diseases caused by phytoplasma and by fastidious vascular-colonizing bacteria, the bacteria reside and multiply within the sieve tube of the phloem, impeding the downward migration of nutrients.
- In tree trunk diseases the pathogen infects the bark and remains attached to the bark for a long time.
- During this time, pathogens attack and destroy phloem elements in this area, affecting nutrient downshift.
- Examples of diseases in which pathogens block the downward movement of organic nutrients
    - White pine blister rust in pine trees whose bark and phloem were killed by the fungus *Cronartium ribicola.*
    - Phytoplasma filling the phloem sieve tubes and restrict the downshift of organic nutrients.
    - Potato tubers with vein necrosis due to potato leaf curl virus.
    - A young rot caused by the fungus Nectoria, where the bark of a branch is attacked and killed by the fungus.
    - Two advanced *Nectria crustaceans* in which both the phloem and most of the xylem were killed by the fungus.

5. Effects of pathogens on host plant respiration

- When a plant is attacked by a pathogen, it generally increases its respiration rate.
- This means that affected tissue depletes carbohydrate stores faster than healthy tissue.
- Increased respiratory rate occurs soon after infection (at least when visible symptoms appear) and continues to increase as the pathogen multiplies and sporulates. Respiration then drops to a normal level, or even lower than that of a healthy plant.
- Respiration increases more rapidly in infections with resistant strains, which require large amounts of energy and are used to rapidly generate

or recruit cellular defense mechanisms. However, in resistant strains, respiration also decreases rapidly after reaching maximum respiration.

- Respiration increases slowly after inoculation, but continues to increase and remains at high levels for much longer periods in susceptible strains that are unable to rapidly recruit defense mechanisms against specific pathogens.
- Some enzymes in the airways appear to have increased activity or concentration.
- Increased respiration in diseased plants is also accompanied by increased activation of the pentose pathway, the major source of phenolic compounds that play an important role in the plant's defense mechanisms against infection.

6. Effect of pathogens on cell membrane permeability

- The cell membrane acts as a permeability barrier, allowing the passage of substances required by the cell into the cell and preventing the passage of substances required by the cell out of the cell.
- Changes in cell membrane permeability are often the first detectable response of cells to infection by pathogens, most toxins, certain pathogenic enzymes, and certain toxic chemicals such as phytochemicals. Example; air pollutants.
- The most frequently observed effect of changes in cell membrane permeability is the loss of electrolytes like small water-soluble ions and molecules from cells.
- When host-pathogen interactions are conflicting and the host remains more resilient, electrolyte leakage occurs much earlier and more frequently than when the host is susceptible and develops widespread symptoms.
- When pathogens directly impact the permeability of cell membranes, they do so via activating certain membrane-bound enzymes like ATPase.ATPases are involved in the movement of $H+$ across the cell membrane by interfering with the processes necessary for membrane maintenance and repair by forming membranes or by breaking down the lipid or protein components of membranes by enzymes produced by the pathogen.

7. Effects of pathogens on transcription and translation

7.1. Effects on transcription

- Some pathogens, especially viruses and fungal pathogens such as rust and powdery mildew, affect the transcriptional processes of infected cells.
- In some cases, pathogens affect transcription by altering the composition, structure, or function of chromatin associated with cellular DNA.
- In some diseases, particularly those caused by viruses, pathogens to make own RNA, use host cell nucleotides and machinery either through their own enzymes or by modifying host enzymes (RNA polymerase) that produce RNA.
- Some diseases increase the activity of ribonucleases (enzymes that break down RNA). This is probably because infected plants produce new types of ribonucleases that are not known to be produced in healthy plants.
- Finally, in some diseases, infected plants, especially resistant plants, appear to contain higher levels of RNA than healthy plants, especially in the early stages of infection.
- It is commonly accepted that higher RNA levels and consequently higher transcription in cells suggest a higher production of compounds involved in plant cells' defence systems.

7.2 Effects of pathogens on translation

- Infected plant tissues often show increased activity of several enzymes, particularly those involved in energy production (respiration) or the production or oxidation of various phenolic compounds, some of which are associated with (defense) reactions to infection.
- Even while some of these enzymes (proteins) may already be present in the cell at the time of infection, many others are generated from the beginning, needing higher transcription and translation activity.
- Increased protein synthesis in infected tissues, observed primarily in pathogen-resistant hosts, reaches its highest levels during the early stages of infection from the first minutes up to 2-20 hours after inoculation.

- Treatment of resistant tissue with protein synthesis inhibitors prior to or during infection reduces resistance to pathogens.
- This interpretation suggests that much of the increased protein synthesis in pathogen-challenged plants reflects increased production of enzymes and other proteins involved in plant defense.

12

Genetics of Resistance

1. Genes and Disease

- When various plants such as rice, wheat, tomato and apple are infected with pathogens and cause disease, pathogens are generally different for each host plant type.
- *Venturia inaequalis*, the fungus that causes apple scab, only affects apples. *Fusarium oxysporum f. sp. lycopersici* which causes tomato wilting, only affects tomatoes and so on.
- It is the presence in the pathogen of one or more genes of pathogenicty, specificity, and virulence to the respective host that enables disease development in the host.
- Pathogen virulence genes are usually specific to one or a few related plants that host the pathogen.
- The genes for gene combinations that make a plant susceptible to a particular pathogen are unique to that one plant species and may be unique to several related plant species.
- All plants also have preformed and induced defenses that provide resistance against most pathogens.
- Specificity explains why pathogens that are toxic to one plant species do not affect other plant species.
- Pathogens contain one or usually more than one virulence gene.
- If the additional new virulence genes required to overcome the effects of the plant's new resistance gene are not included, they cannot infect the plant and the plant remains resistant.
- Therefore, even a new gene for resistance to a pathogen can protect plants carrying it from infection by all or most existing strains of the pathogen for at least months and possibly years.

- When new genes for resistance to pathogens are introduced into plant cultivars and the cultivars are planted in the field, new populations (races) of pathogens are created and new virulence genes are introduced that allow pathogens to attack crops containing the new gene for resistance.
- How did this new population of pathogens acquire new genes of virulence?.
- In most cases the new genes were already present at low concentrations or by mutation, but only in a few of pathogen individuals.
- New genes can arise randomly and abruptly de novo through mutation or rearrangement of the pathogen's genetic material due to ongoing genetic variation in the organism.

2. Genetics of host–pathogen interactions

- referred to as pathogen virulence and host plant resistance genetics.
- Infectious plant diseases are caused by the interaction of at least two organisms, a pathogen and a host plant.
- The characteristics of each of these two organisms are determined by DNA, the genetic material organized into many segments that make up genes.
- Host responses, which are degrees of susceptibility or resistance to various pathogens, are genetic traits.
- Pathogens consist of multitude of races.
- Each race has a different ability to attack certain varieties of plant species, but not other varieties.
- When a variety is inoculated with two appropriately chosen races of a pathogen, the variety is susceptible to one race but resistant to the other.
- This clearly shows that in the first case one race has a genetic trait that allows it to attack plants, while the other does not.
- Conversely, if two of properly selected cultivars of the host plant are inoculated with the same race of the pathogen, one cultivar is susceptible and the other is resistant to the same pathogen.
- This clearly shows that one breed has a genetic trait that allows it to fight off pathogens and maintain resistance, while the other does not.

- If several varieties are separately inoculated with one of several races of the pathogen, one pathogen race may infect one set of varieteis and another races may infect another set of varieties including some that can and some that cannot be infected by the previous race, and so on.

Table: Possible reactions of two (left) and four (right) varieties of a plant to two (left) and four (right) races of a pathogen*

Plant variety	Pathogen race		Plant variety	Pathogen race			
	1	2		1	2	3	4
V_1	–	+	V_1	–	+	+	+
V_2	+	–	V_2	+	–	–	+
			V_3	–	+		+
			V_4	+	–	+	–

*Plus signs indicate susceptible (compatible reaction, infection); minus signs indicate resistant (incompatible reaction, noninfection).

- Studies on the inheritance of resistance versus susceptibility in plants show that single genes control resistance and their absence allows susceptibility.
- Studies on the inheritance of avirulence versus virulence in pathogens show that single genes control avirulence and their absence allows virulence.
- Studies of their interaction show that plant R genes are specific to pathogen avr genes.
- Cultivars with specific resistance genes respond differently to different pathogen races and avirulent genes.
- The progeny of these cultivars respond to the same pathogens in the same way as the parent plant.
- This indicates an inherited trait of resistance or susceptibility to pathogens.
- Similarly, in each variety, the offspring of each pathogen elicit the same effects caused by the parent pathogen.
- This also indicates that the virulence or avirulence nature of the pathogen for a particular variety is also genetically inherited.
- Thus, under favorable environmental conditions, the outcome of infection (susceptibility) or non-infection (resistance) in a host-pathogen combination appears to be predetermined by the genetic material of the host and pathogen.

- The number of genes that determine resistance or susceptibility varies from plant to plant because the number of genes that determine the virulence or avirulence varies from pathogen to pathogen.
- Considerable information exists on the genetics of host-pathogen interactions for several diseases such as potato blight, apple scab and other fungi, powdery mildew, tomato leaf mold, grain blight and rust, and several viral and bacterial diseases.

3. Genetic basis of plant disease resistance

Plant disease resistance is generally divided into:

3.1. **Qualitative resistance**: Controlled by the major R gene.

3.2. **Quantitative resistance**: Controlled by multiple genes with minor effect.

3. 1. Qualitative disease resistance

- The R gene confers complete resistance to a specific pathogen or pathogen strain.
- Easy to operate for basic research and crop improvement.
- Many R genes have been cloned, leading to a better understanding of the downstream responses triggered by R genes.
- Resistance mediated by major R genes can be rapidly overcome by new virulent pathogens.

3.2. Quantitative disease resistance

- Regulated by multiple genes, each contributing to partial resistance.
- Tend to be more persistent than R gene-mediated resistance.
- Reduces selection pressure on pathogen variants.
- Use by conventional or marker-assisted plant breeding methods that yield commercially acceptable levels of disease control.

4. Molecular basis of plant responses to pathogen invasion

- At the molecular level, defense systems often rely on the combination of a particular set of dominant R genes in plants and a corresponding set of dominant non-pathogenic genes (Avr) in pathogens.
- Avr gene expression triggers a plant defense response controlled by the R gene product.

- This gene for gene resistance strategy underlies the molecular basis of plant defense systems.
- This strategy was first proposed by Flor (1955) when studying flax resistance to rust.
- This molecular basis is defined by a single plant R gene against a single pathogen Avr gene, hence the name gene for gene resistance.
- If the plant is resistant, the pathogen is called avirulent and the interaction is called incompatible.
- A pathogen is said to be virulent if the plant is susceptible and the interaction is said to be compatible.
- For a given plant-pathogen interaction, it is often possible for more than one specific combination of Avr and R genes to be activated simultaneously, and such different combinations are often co-dominant.
- These diverse combinations reflect the complexity of plant defense mechanisms during pathogen attack.
- Physiological properties such as K+/H+ exchange, rapid oxidative burst, hypersensitivity at sites of infection, crosslinking of plant cell walls, synthesis of antimicrobial compounds known as phytoalexins, and induction of pathogen-associated proteins such as chitinases and glucanases part of multiple turnover leading to disease resistance.
- The molecular mechanisms underlying the activation of plant defenses are quite different in biotrophs and necrotroph.
- Plant defense against biotrophic pathogens is primarily gene to gene based.
- R gene-mediated resistance usually causes a hypersensitivity reaction (HR).
- It is very important that plants combat biotrophic pathogens such as *Peronospora parasitica*, *Pseudomonas syringae* and *Erysiphe* by limiting access to water and nutrients.
- R gene-mediated resistance also activates SA-dependent signaling, leading to activation of a number of putative defense effector genes.
- This activation of SA signaling occurs throughout the plant and develops systemic acquired resistance (SAR) to subsequent pathogen infection.

5. Gene for Gene hypothesis

- Hypothesis first proposed by HH Flor on flax rust (*Melampsora lini*).
- Latter operate on many other rusts, powdery mildew, apple scab, potato blight and other diseases caused by fungi, various bacteria, viruses, parasitic higher plants and nematodes.

5.1. Concept

- The side-by-side coexistence of host plants and their pathogens in nature indicates that they co-evolved.
- Changes in pathogen virulence appear to be continually offset by changes in host resistance and vice versa.
- In this way, a dynamic balance of resistance and virulence is maintained, allowing both host and pathogen to survive for significant periods of time.
- The stepwise evolution of virulence and resistance can be explained by the gene for gene concept.

5.2. Hypothesis

Each gene that confers virulence to the pathogen there is a corresponding gene in the host that confer resistance to the host and vice versa.

Gene combination and disease reaction types in a host-pathogen system in which gene for gene concept for one gene operates

Generally in host

1. Genes for resistance are dominant –**R**
2. Gene for susceptibility are recessive-**r**

In pathogen

1. Gene for avirulence (inability to infect) are dominant-**A**
2. Gene for virulence are recessive-**a**

Outcome

- Each gene in the host can be identified only by its counterpart gene in the pathogen and vice versa.

Quadratic Check of Gene Combinations and Disease Reaction Types in a Host–Pathogen System in Which the Gene-for-Gene Concept for One Gene Operates*

Virulence or avirulence R (resistant) r (susceptible) genes in the pathogen	Resistance or Susceptibility genes in the plant	
	R (resistant) Dominant	r (susceptible) Recessive
A (avirulent) dominant	AR (-)	Ar (+)
a (virulent) recessive	aR (+)	ar (+)

*Minus signs indicate incompatible (resistant) reactions and therefore no infection.
Plus signs indicate compatible (susceptible) reactions and therefore infection develops.

Gene combination	**Reaction**	**Reason**
AR	Resistant	Host R gene recognizes avirulence gene (A)
Ar	Susceptible	Host lack gene for resistant (R) and so pathogen attack it with other gene of virulence
aR	Susceptible	Although host has gene for resistance (R) pathogen lack gene for avirulence
ar	Susceptible	Plant has no resistance (R) & pathogen is virulent (a)

Complementary interaction of two host genes for resistance and the corresponding two pathogen genes for virulence and their reactions types

Virulence (a) or avirulence (A) genes in the pathogen	Resistance (R) or Susceptibility (r) genes in the plant				
		R_1R_2	$R_1 r_2$	$r_1 R_2$	$r_1 r_2$
	$A_1 A_2$	−	−	−	+
	$A_1 a_2$	−	−	+	+
	$a_1 A_2$	−	+	−	+
	$a_1 a_2$	+	+	+	+

1	Susceptible plant lacking gene for resistance (r_1 r_2) are attacked by all race of the pathogen regardless of the virulence (aa) or avirulence genes (A_1A_2) carried by the pathogen.
2	Pathogen races or individaul designated (a_1a_2), which lack gene for avirulence (A_1A_2) for each gene for resistance of the host (R_1R_2) that infect all plant the have any combination of these genes (R_1R_2, R_1r_2, r_1R_2) since the a_1a_2 pathogen produces no elicitor molecule capable of triggering the host defense.
3	When a pathogen has one of the two genes for virulence (a_1 or a_2) , that is , it lacks one of the two genes of avirulence (A_1 or A_2), then it can infect plants that have corresponding gene for resistance (R_1 or R_2) but not plants that have a gene for resistance corresponding to a gene for avirulence in the pathogen. Ex. Pathogen with A_1a_2 genes infects plant with r_1 R_2 but not those with R_1 r_2, because R_1 can recognize the avr gene A_1 and triggers defenses against it.

6. Nature of resistance to disease

- Resistance adjusted by various internal and external factors.
- They worked to reduce the chances and level of host infection.
- First stage of infection: host recognition by pathogen and vice versa.
- Absence of host recognition factors may help avoid infection by certain pathogens.
- Genetic traits that contribute to plant disease resistance:
    - Pathogen localization and isolation at the point of entry.
    - Reduces the harmful effects of toxic substances produced by pathogens.
    - Inhibits growth and spread of pathogens.

Results

- Pathogens are localized according to varying degrees of invasion and colonization of host tissues.
- In fact, there are very few diseases in which a pathogen freely enters a plant and kills the entire plant.
- Genetic traits that allow a particular variety to complete its life cycle under conditions that do not favor pathogen development also contribute to resistance (DISEASE ESCAPE).

7. Contribution of the genes conditioning resistance in the host

- Genes provide the genetic potential for plants to develop one or more morphological or physiological traits that contribute to disease resistance.
- Production of inducible enzymes or mycotoxic substances required for defense called elicitors.
- Elicitors are secreted by pathogens, react with host cell receptor molecules, and signal other host cell molecules to activate plant defense.
- Conversely, when a mutant pathogen emerges that does not secrete a specific elicitors, the pathogen infects the host without resistance, causing disease and reduced resistance.
- Other potential methods of breaking host resistance are mutations in pathogens that enable them to produce substances that can react with

and neutralize the host's protective toxins directed against them, and removal of the pathogen's protective toxins. or mutations in blocking pathogens. A receptive site in itself that is attacked by the host's defenses.

8. Genetics of resistance through Hypersentsitive response (HR)

- HR is locally self-induced cell death at the site of infection in the host plant in response to infection by pathogens in certain resistant cultivar.
- Whole plant species can be host of pathogens, but individual plant cultivars can be susceptible or resistant to specific race of pathogens.
- Resistance by HR is the result of a gene for gene system in which the pathogen's avirulent gene (avr) corresponds to the host plant's resistance gene (R).
- HR occurs in diseases caused by obligate and facultative pathogens such as viruses, mollicutes, bacteria, fungi and nematodes.

Mechanism

- Recognition by plants of specific signaling molecules, so-called elicitors, produced by the pathogen's avirulent genes and recognized by specific receptor molecules encoded by R genes within the plant.
- Such recognition leads to the activation of host gene cascades leading to hypersensitivity reactions, inhibition of pathogen growth and resistance.
- It also leads to activation of many other defense genes leading to other types of resistance including HR & SAR.

9. Elicitors of defense responses in plants

- Elicitors that initiate plant defense responses.
- Pathogens produce them, and they include a range of molecules.
- Some elicitors are host-specific. i.e. they induce protective responses that confer disease resistance only in specific host varieties.
- An elicitor produced by the avr gene that interacts with the corresponding R resistance gene of the host plant.
- Most elicitors signal the presence of potential pathogens to both host and non-host plants, but some common elicitors are recognized by a minority of plants.

- In nature, the elicitors molecule either reacts directly with the R-encoded receptor protein, releases a compound, or reacts with another host protein (endogenous elicitors) and interacts with the R-encoded receptor.

9.1. General elicitors

Sl.No	Name of Elicitors	Characteristics
1	Harpins	• Produced by numerous gram -ve bacteria . • Part of type III secretion system. • Cause HR and defense gene response.
2	Flagellin	• Produced by gram -ve bacteria . • Part of flagellum. • Cause callose formation and defense gene response.
3	Glycoproteins	• Propuced by Phytophthora. • Induce phytoalexin production and defense gene response.
4	Glycopeptide fragments	• Produced by yeast. • Activate defense genes and ethylene production.
5	Glucans	• Produced by Phytophthora and Pythium. • Derived from oomycete cell wall. • Induce phytoalexins production.
6	Chitin oligomers	• Produced by higher fungi. • Derived from chitin of fungal cell wall. • Induce phytoalexins production and lignifications.
7	Pectin oligomers	• Produced by fungi and bacteria. • Derived from degraded cell wall. • Inhibit proteins and defense genes.
8	Ergosterol	• Produced by various fungi. • Main sterol of higher fungi. • Causes alkalinization in cell cultures.
9	Bacterial toxins	• Such as coronatine of *Pseudomonas syringae*. • Toxin, disturbs salicylic acid. • Mimics jasmonic acid. • Induces defense genes and defense compounds.

10. Avirulence (avr) genes

- Bacterial toxins.
- One of the elicitors of the plant defense response.
- First identified by H.H. Flor in the 1950s.
- The avr gene renders pathogens avirulent.
- Pathogens cannot cause disease in certain types of host plants because their protein products alert plants to the presence and impending attack of pathogens, and host plants mobilize their defenses to block infection by pathogens.

- Thus, the avr gene alerts the host, thereby preventing infection by pathogens.
- Determine the host range of pathogens at the species and race-variety level.

11. Gene coded proteins

Avr protein: Protein coded by pathogen avr genes.

Characteristics of AVR Gene-Coded Protein

- According to the gene-for-gene concept, each dominant gene that affects host plant resistance corresponds to a dominant gene that controls avirulence in the pathogen.
- The elicitor-receptor model, according to which the avirulence (Avr) gene of a pathogen creates an elicitor (Avr) protein that is recognised by a receptor protein expressed by the complementary resistance (R) gene of the host plant, provides the biocchemical or molecular foundation for understanding the gene-for-gene concept.
- The simplest way of confirmation would be if the protein expressed by the host's resistance gene that matched the pathogen's elicitor interacted with it.
- A series of defensive reactions are triggered when the host plant recognises the elicitor protein. These reactions frequently involve cell death around the infection site.
- The hypersensitive response, which is a hallmark of gene-for-gene-based resistance, is the death of cells close to the site of infection.
- When compared to R proteins, Avr proteins, which are encoded by pathogen Avr genes, have less similarities.
- It would appear that in addition to serving as avirulence factors, Avr genes likely serve some other purpose that is advantageous to the pathogen because the majority of Avr genes still persist among a population of pathogens.
- It is now widely acknowledged that the proteins produced by the few Avr genes for which a distinct role for the pathogen has been established have two roles, one of which contributes to the pathogen virulence.
- Avr proteins appear to interact with specific plant proteins known as virulence targets, which are, for example, involved in host metabolism

or plant defence, to contribute to such an effect. Avr proteins' interactions with these targets may increase the pathogen's access to nutrients or dampen the host plant's immune system.

- The only Avr protein for which a biochemical purpose has been precisely established to far is the AvrD protein, which is produced by the AvrD gene of the bacterial spot of tomato pathogen Pseudomonas syringae pv. tomato.
- The AvrD protein performs this role by controlling the production of low molecular weight syringolide elicitors, which cause the soybean to exhibit a hypersensitive response.
- Syringolide-binding proteins have been discovered in resistant soybean plants; these proteins may correspond to the proteins produced by the host plant's R gene.
- Avr proteins, which are produced by pathogen avr genes, appear to share similar characteristics.
- The majority of Avr proteins appear to be hydrophilic, making them water soluble since they lack sequences of hydrophobic amino acids that would allow them to be anchored in cell membranes.
- The "signal sequences" that would enable Avr proteins to be released into the extracellular media via the main secretory route are likewise absent in these proteins.
- Therefore, it would seem that avr gene proteins are generated and either localised in the pathogen cytoplasm or they are released through membrane holes created by Hrp proteins (harpins), which are proteins encoded by the hypersensitive response and pathogenicity (hrp) genes.
- The Avr proteins may directly function as elicitors if they are released externally. The avr gene proteins may function enzymatically to form an elicitor molecule that is carried freely across the bacterial membrane if they are localised in the pathogen cytoplasm.
- In either scenario, the elicitor responds either directly or indirectly with the resulting plant resistance R gene product.

Structures

- Even while avr genes differ greatly, some of them have common structural traits that let us classify avr genes into different families.

- The best known group of avr genes is the *Xanthomonas* avr gene family called ptb genes (for pathogenicity).
- Members of this gene found in Xanthomonas bacteria.
- They produce proteins with between 13 and 23 copies of a nearly identical 34 amino acid repeat unit in their core region.
- Avr/ptb genes cause HR and are also required for the induction of angular leaf spot symptoms in cotton and citrus canker.
- Leaf spots, cankers, and the HR are three quite diverse symptoms that are elicited by one or a few amino acid variations in the repetitive sections of these genes.

12. Function of avr gene proteins

- The avrD gene is found in the bacterium *Pseudomonas syringae* pv.*glycinea.*
- avrCf9 and avrCf4 are contained in tomato leaf mould pathogen *Cladosporium fulvum.*
- Avr gene product of these pathogens is the precursor of the elicitor peptide.
- They are exported and cause HR in hosts with appropriate R genes for resistance.
- An elicitor is located on the coat protein of TMV and causes hypersensitivity reactions to *Nicotiana sylvestris* tobacco, which carries the N gene for resistance.
- In some viral infections, the intracellularly produced viral coat protein appears to act as a specific elicitors to activate the host's HR with their R gene of that virus.

13. Role of avr genes in pathogenicity and virulence

- Most avr genes are not involved in pathogen pathogenicity or virulence.
- Some avr genes, such as the avr-Bs2 gene of the bacterium *Xanthomonas campestris pv.vesicatoria*, encode proteins that are also required for pathogenicity.
- Avr genes like pth A gene from *Xanthomonas citri* and avrb6 for *Xanthomonas campestris pv. malvacearum* , encodes protein that act as pathogencity or virulence factors. They increase the virulence of weakly pathogenic leaf spot strains of *Xanthomonas citrumelo.*

- Pth A is essential for pathogenicity of *Xanthomonas citri* on citrus to cause typical citrus canker disease on host and as avirulence genes , for example by causing pth –A transofrmed strains of *Xanthomonas phaseoli* and *Xanthomonas campestris pv. malvacearum* that, infect beans or cotton , but not citrus, to cause HR on their respective hosts bean and cotton while remaining non pathogenic on citrus.

14. hrp genes

- Referred to as pathogenicity and hypersensitive response genes in bacteria.
- Found primarily in Gram-negative bacteria.
- Additional bacterial genes able to be cause
  - Visible disease on crop hosts.
  - Induces hypersensitivity reactions in certain plants that are not normally infected with bacteria.
  - Allowing bacteria to grow and reach large numbers in susceptible hosts.
  - Several proteins encoded by HRP genes are called harpins and are found in bacterial cell membranes.

15. Other genes involved in pathogenesis and virulence by pathogen

- Pathogenicity factors encoded by pathogenicity genes (pat) and disease-specific genes (dsp) are involved in key steps in disease establishment.
- These genes include essential for:
  - Attachment of pathogens to plant surfaces.
  - Germination and formation of infected structures on the plant surface.
  - Penetration of host.
  - Colonization of host tissue.

16. Resistance (R) genes of plants

- Plant cultivars are resistant to specific pathogen races. This is because plants carry specific resistance genes (R) that allow them to remain resistant to pathogens that have corresponding avirulent genes (avr).

- Many plant R genes and pathogenic Avr genes have been cloned and characterized.
- Another type of her R gene called RPW8 was found in *Arabidopsis thaliana.*
- RPW8 differs in that it confers resistance to a broad range of powdery mildew pathogens rather than specific strains of the pathogen.
- R gene-mediated resistance usually causes a hypersensitivity reaction (HR).

17. How do R gene confer resistance?

- An elicitor molecule produced by the pathogen's avr gene and recognized by a specific plant receptor encoded by the R gene.
- After recognition of the elicitor by the receptor molecule, one or more kinase enzymes are activated and phosphorylation amplifies the signal, which in turn activates other kinases and other enzymes.
- This triggers a cascade of biochemical reactions that lead to HR, resulting in localized host resistance to the pathogen's target.
- Variable SAR values often follow hypersensitivity reactions. These values are represented not only near the attack, but also in certain parts of the plant.

18. Resistance (R) gene of plants

18.1. Hm 1

- The first R gene was isolated in 1991.
- Gene make crop plants resistant to race 1 of the fungus *Cochliobolus miyabeanus (Helminothosporium carbonum)*, which causes maize leaf spot.
- Race 1of *Helminothosporium carbonum* produces a host specific toxin HC-toxin which infect corn variety that lack Hm1 gene and are susceptible to fungus.
- However, race 1 resistant maize cultivars provide expression of the Hm1 gene and produce an enzyme called HC toxin reductase that protects the plant from infection.

18.2. PTO gene

- Confer resistance in tomato to bacterial speck disease caused by *Pseudomonas syringae* pv. *tomato.*
- Pathogen carry avirulence gene avr-pto .
- Protein encoded by the PTO gene appears to be a serine threonine protein kinase, an enzyme suspected play role in HR.

18.3. Cf2, Cf4 &Cf9

- Confer resistance in tomato to leaf mold disease caused by *Cladosporium fulvum* races 2,4 &9 that carry avirulence gene avr2, avr4 &avr9.

18.4. Tobacco N gene

- Confer resistance to TMV virus.

18.5.Flax L6 gene

- Confer resistance to rust fungus *Melampsora lini* race 6 carrying avr6 gene.

18.6. Xa21 gene

- Confer resistance to many races of bacterial leaf blight of rice caused by *Xanthomonas oryzae*

19. Classes of R Genes: According to function

Class	Function	Example of R gene
I	Encodes a detoxifying enzyme	Hm1
II	Encodes a signal transducing protein kinase	PTO
III	Encodes a receptor that transmit signal from protein kinase to phosphokinase for further amplification	Xa21
IV	Encodes cytoplasmic proteins that have a nucleotide binding site and transmit signal to nucleus	N',L6
V	Encodes protein in cytoplasmic membrane that reacts with elicitor product ofavr gene	Cf9

20, Plant defense through R genes and their matching *Avr* genes (Classical Examples)

Predicted structures of known R proteins provide some clues as to how the different protein classes may operate as receptors of *Avr gene products* and as generators and transducers of defense signals.

20.1. Tomato Pto Gene

- Tomato Pto R gene that confers resistance to the bacterium *P. syringae pv. tomato* .
- It encodes a cytoplasmic protein kinase that appears to interact directly with bacterial avrPto proteins that are delivered directly from bacteria to the cytoplasm of plant cells.
- avrPto-mediated hypersensitivity enhanced.
- Expression of Pto requires the presence and expression of another gene, Prf, located within the Pto gene cluster.

20.2. Tobacco N Gene

- A class of cytoplasmic TIR-NBS-LRR R proteins appears in diseases caused by biotrophic fungi, bacteria, viruses, nematodes, and insects.
- All three domains of the N gene protein are required for proper N function.
- In Tobacco mosaic virus (TMV) disease, the viral replicase protein confers avirulence to the virus in cultivars with the N gene and can induce HR in tobacco.
- The N gene encodes the cytoplasmic TIR-NBS-LRR protein.

20.3. Rice Pi-ta Gene

- Rice blast fungus (*Pyricularia oryzae*) has avr-Pi-ta avirulence gene, which is effective on rice cultivars with Pi-ta resistance gene.
- Pi-ta encodes a cytoplasmic protein containing an NBS domain and a leucine-rich carboxyl terminus.
- A direct interaction between the Avr-Pita protein and the leucine-rich domain of Pita was demonstrated.
- This is the first experimental evidence that the AVR protein directly interacts with its R protein. A predicted protease activity of AVR pita is required for its avirulent function.

20.4. Tomato Cf Genes

- In the tomato leaf mold disease, caused by a fungus *Colletotrichum fulvum* carrying any of the genes Avr2, Avr4, or Avr9 confer avirulence to tomato plants carrying the matching resistance R genes Cf2, Cf4, or Cf9.

- *Avr2* encodes an extracellular cysteine-rich protein that is secreted by the fungus during growth in the apoplastic space of tomato leaves.
- As these genes are more than 90% genetically identical, they seem to activate the same defense signaling pathway after the elicitor is recognized

20.5. Tomato Bs2 Gene

- The AvrBs2 of *Xanthomonas campestris* pv. *vesicatoria* on pepper and a number of avr proteins generated by different pathovars of Pseudomonas syringae on their specific hosts are among the most researched bacterial avr proteins to date.
- In the *Xanthomonas campestris pv. vesicatoria* pepper combination, the Bs2 gene codes for an NBS-LRR protein that has a hydrophobic N terminus.
- In addition to conferring resistance to peppers with the Bs2 R gene, the avrBs2 gene, which was shown to be highly conserved among different strains of *Xanthomonas campestris pv vesicatoria* and among other pathovars of *Xanthomonas campestris,* is needed for full virulence of the bacterium on susceptible hosts.

20.6. Arabidopsis RPM1 Gene

- avrRpm1 gene of *Pseudomonas syringae pv. maculicola* confers avirulence to the bacterium on pea, bean, soybean, and arabidopsis .
- Recognition of the AvrRpm1 in arabidopsis requires the presence of the RPM1 gene.
- The RPM1 gene also confers resistance to *Pseudomonas syringae pv. glycinea* expressing the avrB gene.
- These sequences of AvrRpm1 and AvrB are required for the expression of full virulence and for localization of these proteins at the plasma membrane of the host cell.

21. Oligogenic and Polygenic resistance to disease

- Plant pathologists commonly divide resistance into monogenic and polygenic resistance.
- Monogenic resistance is governed by one gene and polygenic resistance

is governed by many genes.

- Gene in monogenic resistance is identified individually by letters or numbers or both.
- Thus the gene R_1 gives the potato resistance to blight, the gene Sr_6 gives wheat and the B gives oats resistance to stem rust.
- It can be determined what sort of resistance the gene gives; whether it is dominant or recessive.
- The gene can be located on some particular chromosome; the gene Sr_6 is on chromosome XX of wheat.
- Inheritance of polygenic resistance is more vague.
- Polygenic resistance is conferred by too many genes to be counted and identified individually.
- No single gene has an effect large enough to be followed or for the gene to be identified and located. One knows only the combined effect of genes as a whole.
- The division of resistance into monogenic and polygenic resistance is popular among plant pathologists when they think in terms of genes, but it is incomplete.
- It makes no rooms for immediate sorts , digenic or trigenic resistance, for example, which are neither monogenic nor polygenic.
- The proper opposite of poly-, meaning many, is oligo-mening few; and if wishes to classify resistance in terms of numbers of genes , one should write of oligogenic rather than monogenic resistance as the opposite of polygenic resistance.
- Digenic resistance of the potato to blight , as in the variety vertifolia with genes R_3 and R_4 and Trigenic resistance as in the variety Greta with the genes $R_{1,}$ $R_{3,}$ and R_4, closely resemble monogenic variety , as in the variety Kennebec with the gene $R_{1.}$

22. Major and Minor gene resistance

- The term major and minor are sometimes used instead of oligogenic and polygenic where referring to gene resistance.
- The system is not without merit, but it probably to be avoided since it might be misleading.

- All oligogenes are not necessarily major genes in the sense of being important genes.
- For example, although, the gene R_1 governing resistance to potato blight merits being called a major gene because it is a strong gene much used in potato breeding, the gene R_4 is a weak and little importance to potato breeders.
- In contrary, all polygenes are not minor genes in the sense being relatively unimportant.
- For example, it is polygenes that have been given maize most of its wide resistance to disease.

23. Vertical and Horizontal resistance

- When a variety is more resistance to some races of a pathogen than to other the resistance is called vertical or perpendicular resistance.
- When resistance is evenly spread against all races of the pathogen, it is called horizontal resistance or lateral resistance.
- VR implies a differential interaction between varieties of host and races of the pathogen. In HR there is no differential interaction.
- It is generally conceded that more resistance genes in the host , the less likely the pathogen is to match them.
- Monogenic resistance on the basis of this argument , can be relatively easily matched, and is therefore more likely to be vertical and overcome by new races of the pathogen.
- The argument is plausible but does not fit the facts well.
- On the other hand, numerous examples are known of monogenic resistance which has survived unscathed over the years and so far as the evidence now goes, seems safe.
- The general argument that resistance given by many genes is safer than resistance given by a few genes is probably sound good, but only when other things are equal.
- Among the other things that may not be equal is the balance between parasitism and saprophytism in the pathogen.
- For example, *Phytophthora infestans* is essentially a parasite, only a slight extent a saprophyte; *Periconia circinata* seems to be almost pure saprophyte .

- Between the two are many grades in the balance between parasitism and saprophytism which affect the stability of resistance.

24. Inheritance of virulence and aggresiveneness

- This is about inheritance in the pathogen, not the host.
- Virulence seems often to be inherited oilgogenically, aggressiveness polygenically.
- Difference between races is quantitative rather than qualitative.
- Pathogenicity includes both aggresivenss and virulence.
- All races of a pathogen are pathogenic.
- There is no evidence for positive correlation between aggresivenss and virulence.
- But there is a negative correlation: Increased virulence may go with decreased aggresivenes.

25. How is resistance translated into a useful effect

25.1. Vertical resistance

- VR delays the start of an epidemic.
- This is only known beneficial effect of R genes.
- They do not slow down the epidemic after it has started.
- They donot reduce the infection rate.
- VR decreases as more virulent races are present.
- The main reason for virulent races becoming abundant is the extensive planting of resistant varieties.
- Farmers who plant more resistant varieties run the risk of destroying much of the resistance and therefore defeating the purpose of developing varieties.
- The increasing popularity of a variety among farmers can be self destructive process when the popularity depends on VR.

25.2. Horizontal resistance

- Slow down the epidemic after it has started
- The delay in start of an epidemic brought about vertical resistance is inversely proportional to the infection rate.

- It is related to the proportion of virulent races in the population of the pathogen.
- Because they affect VR and are themselves affected by HR , infection rates are integral part of resistance theory.

26. Use of resistance

- The first requirement is for resistance genes that are adequate for their task.
- The primary concern in breeding for resistance has always been the availability of desirable genes.

26.1. Resistance to non obligate parasites

- Breeding for resistance is easy when the saprophytic phase is long, as it is in soil-borne diseases of annual crops cultivated in long rotations.
- If genes for resistance can be found, they can be used without further ado.
- If resistance is horizontal, there will be no complications from new races of the pathogen.
- If it is vertical, new races may appear quickly if the genes are weak or moderately weak, as they are in resistance to flax , wilt , or slowly if the genes are as strong as the gene I for resistance to Fusarium wilt of tomatoes or perhaps never, If the gene are very strong.
- But stabilizing selection will persist, weakly or strongly according to the strength of resistance genes.
- The value of the resistance, small if the gene are weak and great if they are strong, is unlikely to be lost by mismanagement, in a way that vertical resistance to obligate parasites can be lost by mismanagement.

26.2. Obligate and No obligate parasite

26.2.1. Host-Host –Pathogen systems

26.2.2. Saprophytic medium- Host –Pathogens systems

- Any plant is susceptible to inoculum coming from a diseased plant of same variety (and the same age), provided that environmental conditions allow disease to occur.
- A plant cannot be genetically resistant to a pathogen that can attack other plants of the same genotype in the same environmental conditions.

- This truism implies that adequate vertical resistance to obligatory parasites can develop only if the epidemic area contains at least two host genotypes; that is, there must be a host-host-pathogen system.
- The resistant variety must have at least one gene that the other host variety lacks.
- If the gene is strong enough, stabilizing selection will act against virulent races. It will prevent virulent races able to match this gene from becoming common on the variety without the gene.
- Unnecessary virulence reduces the fitness of race to survive.
- The essence of this host-host-pathogen system is that the pathogen must move from the variety without the resistance gene to the variety with it.
- This movement may come about for several reasons;
    - The pathogen cannot survive all the year round on the resistant variety.
    - Or the movement may come about because the variety with resistant gene is uncommon, and the variety without it common. The movement remains important only for as long as the acreage of the new vriety remains relatively small.
    - Or the movement may come about when a multiline grown, because in a multiline the pathogen moves from one host genotype to another.
    - All this host true for obligate or near obligate parasites.
- If the pathogen is not an obligate parasite, but has a saprophytic as well as parasitic life, the system is changed.
- For VR to be stable, it is still necessary for the pathogen to reach the resistant variety for an outside source, but the source is now the soil or crop residues or wherever the pathogen spends its saprophytic life.
- With the obligate parasites it is the other variety –the variety without resistant gene – that stabilizes the races and hence the VR.
- The change is from a host-host-pathogen system to a saprophytic medium – host-pathogen system.
- A single host genotype can have VR against a pathogen that is also a saprophyte.

27. Parasitism/Sprophytism

- Parasitism and saprophytism differ in essential processes, and the more specialized as parasite becomes, the more it loses its saprophytic processes.
- The ability to survive saprophytically declines as the ability to parasitize rises.
- Incresed virulence may or may not greatly affect the pathogens ability to survive saprophytically.
- It depends on the strength of the gene that the increased virulence matches; the stronger the gene, the more the pathogens ability to survive saprophytically is affected.
- Gene strength determines the relative ability of the complementary race of the pathogen to survive outside the plant with the gene.

28. Vertical Resistance : Qualitative effect on vertical popularity

- In some (though not all) circumstances virulent races increase in abundance as the resistant varieties that they attack increase in popularity.
- Example: As resistant wheat varieties increased in acreage in Australia, so did the races of *Puccinia grminis* that could attack them.
- The varieties left the breeders nurseries as resistant, because races able to attack them were not known.
- Within a few years they were susceptible, because races able to attack them became abundant. This is the essence of the boom and bust cycle of variety production.
- The relative abundance of virulent races is proportional to the relative acreage of the resistant variety.
- The popularity of a variety is the greatest destroyer of the variety's vertical resistance.
- A plant breeder is in a ludicrous position. He hopes his new variety will become popular among farmers.
- He hopes it will maintain its resistance and hopes are likely to be mutually exclusive.
- These remarks hold only for pathogens that can maintain themselves the year sound on the variety or self sown.

29. Vertical Resistance : Enhancing effect of HR

- An abundance of adequately virulent races is merely one factor in VR. Another consideration is the infection rate.
- Fast infection rates decrease the efficiency of VR; slow rate increase it.
- Weather is one of the factors influencing the infection rate.
- Weather which favours disease raises the rate and diminishes the efficiency of VR; weather that is unfavourable to disease decreases the rate and increases the efficiency.
- HR is more important in this particular instance.
- HR is more important in this particular instance.
- HR reduced the infection rate and thereby enhances VR.
- The good results obtained by combining VR &HR are important to know. The literature of resistance to disease contains much argument about whether VR or HR should be used and discuss the two kinds of resistance as alternatives.
- It seldom recognizes that the two kind are best used in combination- that the one helps the other.

30. Comparison of Vertical resistance & Horizontal resistance

30.1. Vertical resistance

- Resistance conferred by R genes manifests itself as hypersensitivity.
- Race are virulent because they use metabolic pathways that do not provoke a hypersensitive reaction in place of the normal metabolic pathways of virulent races that do provoke a hypersensitive reaction.
- On varieties lacking R genes, altered metabolic pathways are less efficient than normal.
- The virulent gene operates on less efficient parasitic pathways; they are less aggressive on varieties without R genes.
- Resistance will be vertical even in the absence of hypersensitivity.
- VR includes more than just hypersensitivity.

30.2. Horizontal resistance

- Resistance takes the form of resting penetration by the germ tubes of spores before the pathogen can establish itself within the host.

- This type of resistance appears to be common, and host varieties vary greatly in it.
- Resistance to penetration by germ tubes can be matched by spores of the pathogen with higher capacity for spores to germinate; races often vary widely in this.
- Thus resistance that halved the proportion of germ tubes able to penetrate would be matched by a race with spores having double the capacity to germinate.
- If germination and penetration are independent processes and other things are equal , one could rank races for ggresiveness in the order of the capacity of their spores to germinate, which would be independent of the resistance of the host to penetration; and one would rank varieties of the host in order of the spore to germinate.
- When the ranking of races for aggressiveness is independent of the resistance of the varieties for resistance is independent of the aggressiveness of the races, the resistance is horizontal.
- If new race of the pathogen has increased aggressiveness on one variety it has also increased aggressiveness on all other varieties- if , e.g., in overcoming resistance the pathogen becomes more aggressive not only on resistant varieties but also on susceptible varietiether test of ranking is satisfied, and resistance is horizontal

31. Use of multilines

- Multiline is grown from a mixture of seed of different varieties or lines.
- These lines are uniform in all the features that matter agronomically- they are of same height, mature at the same time, etc- but differ in the vertical resistance genes they have.
- Multiline, although they use vertical resistance, have features that make them a substitute for HR.
- HR's benefit to obligate or near-obligate parasites is enormous. A stable host-pathogen system requires only one genotype, whereas efficient VR requires at least two host genotypes in a host host-pathogen system.
- A multiline has several host genotypes, and a stable multiline pathogen system requires just one multiline.
- A multiline pathosystem is really a host-host-pathogen system and for all practical purposes it compares with the simple host-pathogen system of HR.

13

Genetic Variation in Pathogens

Genetic variations

- Genetic variation is the presence of differences in gene sequences between individual organisms of a species.
- Enables natural selection, one of the major forces driving the evolution of life.
- When an individual's offspring exhibit mutations in the traits of their parents, such offspring are called variants.

Importance of variation in plant pathogens

- Diversity in different organisms is a common feature and a critical process for the continuation of life under stressful conditions.
- Plant pathogens especially fungi, bacteria, viruses and nematodes, exhibit variations in virulence and physiological functions that support survival under different environmental conditions.
- These variations may be primarily due to genetic and environmental factors.
- Various studies of the genetic variability of plant pathogens result in mutations in traits that affect their ability to infect host plants and other traits that do not alter virulence but may affect survival.
- Knowledge of virulence trait variation is valuable in planning effective disease control interventions.

Mechanisms of variability

There are two mechanisms of variability in pathogens

I. General mechanisms of variability

II. Specialized mechanisms of variability

Sl.No	General mechanisms of variability	Specialized mechanisms of variability
1	Mutation	Heterokaryosis
2	Recombination	Parasexualism
3	Sexual reproduction	Heteroploidy
4		Conjugation
5		Transformation
6		Transduction
7		Genetic recombination

Different mechanisms of variability in plant pathogens

Sl.No	Fungi	Bacteria	Virus
1	Mutation	Conjugation	Attenuation
2	Recombination	Transformation	Mutation
3	Hybridization	Transduction	Recombination
4	Parasexuality		Selection pressure
5	Heterokaryosis		
6	Hetreoploidy		
7	Adaptation		
8	Saltation		

I. General mechanisms of variability

- Two mechanisms of variability occur in pathogens.

  1. Mutation
  2. Recombination

1. Mutation

1.1 Definition

- A mutation is a more or less sudden change in the genome of an organism.
- It is then genetically passed on to offspring.

1.2 General mechanism of mutation

- Mutations represent changes in the base sequence of DNA .
  - Replace one base with another.
  - Addition or removal of one or more base pairs.
  - Amplification of a specific DNA segment into multiple copies.
  - Insertion or removal of transposable elements.

- Inversion of a DNA segment.
- An average fungal genome consists of approximately 10,000 genes.
- One in 100 fungal cells may be mutants.
- Mutations at loci encoding enzymes can result in alleles that produce altered forms of the enzyme, often called allozymes.
- Mutations occur naturally in all organisms in nature.
- Mutation occurs in those who reproduce both sexually and asexually, and in those who reproduce only sexually or asexually.

1.3. Variability through mutation in plant pathogen

- Mutations in protozoa, bacteria and fungi with haploid mycelium and in viruses can appear shortly after development.
- Most mutations are usually recessive.
- Pathogenic mutations are likely to occur frequently and large numbers of pathogenic mutants differing from their parents are produced in nature each year.
- When a new virulence factor appears in the mutant, it may participate in sexual or quasi-sexual processes in the pathogen and generate recombinants whose degree or type of virulence is quite different from that present in the parental strain.
- Pathogens contain genetic material (DNA) outside the cell nucleus in the form of organelles, plasmid DNA, and even double-stranded RNA.
- Extranuclear DNA mutations are as common as nuclear DNA mutations and affect all properties controlled by extranuclear DNA.
- Inheritance of traits controlled by extranuclear DNA (cytoplasmic inheritance) does not follow Mendelian laws of genetics.
- Due to mutations in extrachromosomal DNA, many pathogens gain or lose the ability to carry out physiological processes that they were previously unable to carry out.
- Cytoplasmic inheritance most likely occurs in all organisms except viruses and viroids, which lack cytoplasm.
- Three types of adaptations driven by changes in cytoplasmic genetic material have been demonstrated in pathogens.

- Develop the ability to tolerate toxic substances.
- Use new substances for growth.
- Alters virulence to host plants.

2. Recombination

- Recombination occurs primarily during sexual reproduction in plants, fungi and nematodes.
- Two haploid (1N) nuclei containing different genetic material at many locations join to form a diploid (2N) nucleus called a fertilized egg.
- The zygote undergoes meiosis to produce new haploid gametes.
- Recombination of different genes or alleles of the same gene occurs during meiosis of the fertilized egg as a result of genetic mating.
- Recombination occurs in the fertilized egg and the haploid nuclei or gametes obtained after meiosis are different from each other than the gametes that produced the zygote.
- Recombination can also occur during mitotic cell division during individual development and is involved in important gene exchanges in fungi.
- In fungi, haploid nuclei or gametes often undergo mitosis to produce haploid mycelium and spores, which are relatively homogenous individuals that can produce large asexual populations by the next life cycle, yields a genetically distinct group of.

2.1 Gene and genotypic flow among plant pathogens

- Gene flow is the process by which specific alleles (genes) move from one population to another geographically diverse population.
- Gene flow is very important in plant pathology. Gene flow is about the transmission of pathogenic mutant alleles between different field populations.
- A pathogen's high gene flow increases the population and geographic area in which its genetic material is found.
- In general, pathogens with high gene flow have higher genetic diversity than pathogens with low gene flow.
- In plant pathogens that reproduce only asexually, recombination does not occur and entire genotypes can be transferred between populations. This is called genotype flow.

- Pathogens that produce resting spores and other forms of growth. For examples long-range rusts and powdery mildews, their genomes are wide and can sometimes spread across continents.
- Soil-borne fungi and nematodes are slow-moving, localized, and have limited gene flow.
- Pathogens with high gene or genotype flow are much more effective than pathogens with low gene flow and pose a greater threat to agriculture.
- Asexual spores and reproductive organs already contain a set of fully adapted and selected alleles. Such reproductive organs are at higher risk of extended coverage due to genotypic flow than sexual reproductive organs due to gene flow.

2.2. Genetic drift among plant pathogens

- The populations of most organisms in a geographic area may not be large enough to ensure that each variant will be passed on to the next generation, so random effects may occur during the transmission of genetic traits to new generations will occur. This is called random genetic drift.
- In plant pathology, pathogens occurring in large populations have greater evolutionary potential than pathogens occurring in small populations.
- Larger populations increase the likelihood that new, more fit mutants will emerge within the host, can multiply within the host, and spread to new hosts before mutations are lost through genetic drift.
- Cultivation practices and chemical management that regularly slash field pathogen populations are less diverse and adapt much slower than populations that can sustain high populations throughout the year.

2.3. Selection of plant pathogens

- Selection is a directional process in which variants that are most suitable for a particular environment increase their frequency in the population (positive selection) and less suitable variants decrease their frequency (negative selection).
- As a result of selection in populations large enough for all variants to be passed on to the next generation.
- Variant frequencies at equilibrium provide an estimate of the goodness of fit of the variant.

- Selection leads to less diversity within populations, but can lead to more diversity between populations.

2.4 Life Cycles

- The life cycle is very simple and is predominantly asexual in bacteria and oomycetes.
- They may include strictly haploid life cycles, haploid-dikaryotic life cycles, haploid-diploid, diploid, or asexual life cycles.
- The outcross life cycles of different plant pathogens vary greatly.
- Most complex in some oomycetes and fungi.
- The nature of the life cycle and subsequent mating system influence the genetic diversity and evolutionary opportunities and limits of individual pathogens.
- Example; the wheat stem rust fungus *Puccinia graminis* f. sp *tritici*. In the haploid state, it infects barberry, and in the diploid state, it infects wheat.
- Genotypic diversity is more important than genetic diversity in asexual pathogen populations.
- Genetic diversity is more important than genotypic diversity in sexual pathogen populations.
- Therefore, a pathogen that undergoes some type of recombination poses a greater threat than a pathogen that undergoes little or no recombination.
- Recombinant pathogen populations can assemble new combinations of virulence genes or alleles as fast as breeders can assemble resistance genes.
- Pyramiding resistance genes into plants may not be as effective a strategy as plant breeders hoped.
- Outbred pathogens that produce more new genotypes pose a greater threat to crops than inbred pathogens.

Pathogen Fitness

- Fitness is the ability of pathogens to survive and multiply.
- Pathogen fitness can be quantified by measuring its fecundity, multiplication rate, efficiency of infection, and aggressiveness.

- Fitness appears to be the driving force behind the stability and development of pathological systems in agriculture.
- Specific interactions between pathogens with avirulence genes and hosts with resistance-adapted R genes, mutations to virulence occur to increase pathogen fitness while the R gene is present.

Specialized mechanisms of variability in fungi

1.1. Parasexualism

- Parasexuality in fungi can be explained as genetic recombination without meiosis.
- Fungi exist and grow primarily as adjacent hyphae that form heterokaryons as a result of anastomosis or fertilization.
- Parasexuality is the process by which genetic recombination can occur within fungal heterokaryons.
- Therefore, the genetic diversity resulting from parasexualism may equal or exceed that achieved through sexual reproduction.
- This is caused by the occasional fusion of two nuclei to form a diploid nucleus.
- During proliferation, several mitotic crossovers lead to the appearance of the recombinant as a diploid cell nucleus.
- The diploid nucleus gradually loses a single chromosome and reverts to the haploid state.
- Parasexuality has been reported in many rust fungi, including *Puccinia graminis tirtici, Puccinia coronata* and some smut, *Ustilago hordei* and *Ustilago maydis.*

1.2 Heterokaryosis

- The phenomenon of different types of cell nuclei in the same individual is called heterokaryosis.
- Hansen and Smith (1932) first proposed heterokaryosis as his remedy, a variation of *Botrytis cinerea.*
- A condition in which a fungal hypha or some cells of a hypha contain two or more nuclei that are genetically distinct as a result of fertilization or anastomosis.

- For example, in basidiomycetes, the dikaryotic state can differ significantly from the haploid mycelium and spores of fungi.
- In *Puccinia graminis tritici*, the causative agent of wheat stem rust, haploid basidiospores infect barberry but not wheat and haploid mycelium can only grow on barberry. However, dikaryotic aeciospores and uredospores can infect wheat but not barberry. Dikaryotic mycelium can grow on both barberry and wheat.
- Pathogenicity is also influenced by heterokaryosis, demonstrated in *Fusarium oxysporum f. pisi,* the causative agent of pea wilting.
- Heterokaryosis also occurs in many sac fungi, basidiomycetes, and imperfect fungi.

1.3. Heteroploidy

- The presence of cells, tissues, or whole organisms in which the number of chromosomes per nucleus differs from the organism's normal 1N or 2N complementarity.
- Heteroploids can be haploid, diploid, triploid or tetraploid, or they can be aneuploid (e.g. 2n-1) or euploid (e.g. N + 1).
- Heteroploids is often associated with cell differentiation and is a normal developmental situation in most eukaryotes.
- Heteroploids have been shown to affect the color, enzymatic activity, and pathogenicity in fungi. Aneuploids lose the ability to infect cotton, even when derived from highly virulent haploids.
- Example, some heteroploids, such as diploids of the normally haploid fungus *Verticillium alboatrum*, the cause of wilt in cotton, lose the ability to infect cotton plants even when derived from highly virulent haploids.

1.4. Vegetative Incompatibility

- In some fungi, the vegetative hyphae of the same colony or two colonies of the same species come into contact with each other and often fuse. The fusion is called a mycelial anastomosis.
- However, if the contacting hyphae do not belong to different strains, but belong to the same species, hyphal fusion will not occur, resulting in trophic (or somatic or heterokaryotic) incompatibility.
- In some filamentous fungi, such as the species *Thanatephorus cucumeris*, a teleomorph of *Rhizoctonia solani*, fusion incompatibility occurs

between distantly related strains that appear to be different species, leading to trophic and sexual fusion both are hindered, does not allow the exchange of genetic material.

- Various fusion incompatibility groups may represent different yet unrecognized species within the broader species of *Thanetophorus cucumeris.*
- When hyphae from two colonies belonging to different post-fusion incompatibility groups meet, the hyphae fuse, but then the cytoplasm of the two combined hyphal compartments and some adjacent compartments is disrupted, A sparse and sometimes dark border zone of mycelium is produced.
- Such post-fusion incompatibility is the result of interaction between two alleles of the same trophic compatibility locus (v-c) and is called allelic incompatibility.
- Nutrient incompatibility appears to be a defense mechanism that protects individuals from harmful nuclei, mitochondria, plasmids, and viruses that may reach individuals from other cells through anastomoses.

1.5. Adaptation

- A pathogen becomes adapted when it acquires the ability to carry out a physiological process that it was previously unable to carry out or could not carry out efficiently.
- This phenomenon is known as adaptation.
- Pathogenicity adaptations for Fusarium, Phytophthora, and *Helminthsporium* spp.

1.6. Saltation

- Salting is represented by morphologically distinct regions or sectors of fungal colonies. These sectors can remain stable or salted again.
- Saltation is found in the genera Fusarium, Helminthsporium, Alternaria and Sphaceroteca.

2. Mechanisms of Variability in Bacteria

Variability in bacteria seem to arise by means of

2.1. Vertical gene transfer

- The transfer of genetic information in this manner is not always limited to members of the same species or even genus.

2.1.1. Conjugation

- Two compatible bacteria come into contact with each other.
- Small portions of chromosomes or plasmids are transferred from one bacterium to another via conjugative bridges or pili.
- Conjugation is a form of genetic recombination.
- Genetic recombination refers to the process that results in the formation of new individuals whose genes are partly derived from one parent and partly from another genetically distinct parent.
- Conjugation increases the genetic diversity of bacterial populations and facilitates the emergence of antibiotic resistance.

2.1.2. Transformation

- No cell contact required.
- Bacterial cells are genetically transformed by assimilating into their own cells genetic material that is shed by other bacteria or released during decomposition.
- This is the method used to induce mutations by recombination in the laboratory.
- It is also found in the natural world.

2.1.3. Transduction

- No cell contact required
- Bacterial viruses (phages) transfer genetic material from the bacterium in which the phage was produced to the next infecting bacterium.
- Such transmission of genetic information is not always restricted to members of the same species or genus.
- This process creates a new genotype of the bacterium.

2.2. Horizontal gene transfer

- Gram-negative bacteria can easily transfer genetic material between species.
- Agrobacterium transfers genes to plants across regional barriers.
- Such events are called horizontal gene transfer.

3. Mechanisms of variability in viruses

3.1. Genetic recombination

- Inoculation of two strains of the same virus into the same host plant will yield one or more new virus strains with different properties than the original two strains introduced into the host.
- New strains are likely to be recombinant, but we cannot always exclude the occurrence by mutation rather than hybridization.
- For multipartite viruses consisting of two, three or more nucleic acid components, new strains of virus can be introduced into host plants or vectors by recombination of the corresponding components of two or more strains of such virus.

3.2. Mutation

- Mutations are also an important source of mutants.
- Mutations include base substitutions and deletion mutations.
- Base substitutions lead to point mutations that change the base of a nucleotide in a way that the parent protein molecule encodes.
- Such base substitutions were found in cauliflower mosaic virus and tobacco mosaic virus.
- Deletion mutations occur when part of the genome is deleted and the mutant loses the characters encoded by the deleted genome segment.
- Deletion mutations were first reported in wound tumor viruses by Reddy and Black (1974, 1977).
- Mutations have been found in several other viruses since the deletion.

3.3. Selection pressure

- Selection pressure leading to selection of new strains under altered conditions.
- The previously dependent strain in the mixture becomes the new dominant strain when the selection pressure shifts, which seems to promote the formation of new strains.
- Temperature and host are two of the most common and important selection pressures in nature, leading to the selection of new strains.

3.4 Attenuation

- Attenuation means partial or complete loss of virulence of the virus.
- Attenuation also increases the genetic diversity of the virus population.
- It also facilitate the emergence of new strains/biotypes.

4. Stages of variation in pathogens

4.1. Species

- The total population of a particular organism on earth. eg. a fungal pathogen that shares certain common morphological and other phenotypic characteristics and forms pathogenic species.
- Example: *Puccinia graminis,* the causative agent of cereal stem rust.

4.2. Varieties or Special forms

- However, some individuals of this species live exclusively on wheat, barley, or oats, and these individuals form groups known as varietals or special forms (*Formae specialis*).
- Examples: *Puccinia graminis tritici, Puccinia graminis hordei and Puccinia graminis avenae*

4.3. Race

- Even within each special form, however, some individuals attack some of the varieties of the host plant but not others, some attack another set of host plant varieties, and so on, with each group of such individuals making up a race.
- Examples: There are more than 200 races of *Puccinia graminis tritici* (race 1, race 15, race 59, and so on).

4.4. Variant

- Occasionally, one of the offspring of a race can suddenly attack a new variety or can cause severe symptoms on a variety that it could barely infect before.
- This individual is called a variant.

4.5 Biotype

- The identical individuals produced asexually by the variant make up a biotype.
- Each race consists of one or several biotypes (race 15A, 15B, and so on).

14

Disease Control by Immunization

Introduction

- Most common improvement of host resistance to almost any pathogen is brought about by improving the genetic resistance of the host, that is by breeding and using resistance varieties.
- Genetic engineering technology made possible the isolation of individual resistance (R) genes from resistant plants and the transfer of such genes into susceptible plants in which they induce the hypersensitive resistant response.
- Thus, genetic engineering technology combined with Conventional plant breeding, will provide one of the most effective tools for controlling plant diseases.
- Inoculation of plants with certain pathogens often leads to temporary or nearly permanent immunization of the plants, that is, induced plant resistance to a pathogen to which the plants are normally susceptible .
- Some of these treatments involve only viruses and are known as cross protection; others may involve different kind of pathogens and are known as induced or systemic acquired resistance.
- Inoculation of plants with certain pathogens often leads to temporary or nearly permanent immunization of the plants, that is, induced plant resistance to a pathogen to which the plants are normally susceptible.

1. Cross protection

Protection of a plant by a mild strain of viruses from infection by a strain of the same viruses that causes more severe symptoms.

Application

- Controlling viral diseases.
- Tomatoes with mild strains of Tobacco mosaic virus.
- Citrus with mild strains of Citrus tristeza virus.
- Papaya with mild strains of Papaya ring spot virus.

Limited use in crop protection

Cross protection has not gained wide spread use due to

- Non availability of appropriate mild strains of viruses.
- Mild strains are not effective against all severe strains present in different localities.
- Method for field crops is laborious.
- Danger of mutation toward new more virulent strains and spread to other crops.
- Crop protection ability of mild strain is lost after few years.

2. Defense through plantibodies

- Plants, donot have an immune system like that of humans and animals, that is, they donot produce antibodies.
- Of late, transgenic plants have been produced that have been genetically engineered to incorporate in their genome, and to express, foreign genes, such as mouse genes that produce antibodies against certain pathogens.
- Such antibodies, encoded by animal genes but produced in and by the plant, are called plantibodies.
- Transgenic plants producing plantibodies against coat proteins of viruses, For example, artichoke mottle crinkle virus, to which they are susceptible, can defend themselves and show some resistance to infection by these viruses.
- This type of plant immunization will yield great dividends by expressing in plants animal antibody genes that will produce antibodies directed against specific essential proteins of the pathogen *viz*., viral replicases or movement proteins and fungal and bacterial enzymes of attack.

3. Induced resistance

Inoculation of plants with certain pathogens often leads to temporary or nearly permanent immunization of the plants, that is, induced plant resistance to a pathogen to which the plants are normally susceptible .

Resistant to pathogens could be induced in their hosts by

- Treating the host with naturally occurring compounds obtained from the pathogen.
- Treating hosts with unrelated natural compounds.

3.1. Treating the host with naturally occurring compounds obtained from the pathogen;

- Coat protein of TMV.
- Proteinaceous component or glycoprotein fraction from a bacterium (*Pseudomonas solanacearum*).
- Lipid component from a fungus(*Phytophthora infestans*).
- Polysaccharide such as chitosan from a fungus.

3.2. Treating hosts with unrelated natural compounds;

- Water soluble fraction of non pathogenic bacterium.
- Polysaccharide from a nonpathogenic fungus.
- Proteinaceous compounds isolated from an unrelated plant.

Examples

1. Bean and sugarbeet inoculated with virus exhibit a greater resistance to infection by certain obligate fungal pathogens causing rusts and powdery mildews than do virus free plants.
2. In tobacco, TMV induces a systemic resistance not only to itself but also to unrelated viruses, to fungi like *Phytophthora nicotianae*, to bacteria like *Pseudomonas tabaci* and even to certain aphids.
3. Inoculation of tobacco with fungi *viz.*, *Chalara elegans* (*Thielaviopsis basicola*) or a bacterium *viz.*, *Pseudomonas syringae* induces systemic resistance to TMV.
4. Inoculation of apple with nonpathogenic bacterium induces resistance against fire blight of apple.

4. Local and Systemic acquired resistance

1. Induced resistance is at first localized around the point of plant necrosis, caused by infection by the pathogen or by the chemical is called local acquired resistance (LAR).
2. Subsequently, resistance spread systematically and develops in distal, untreated parts of the plant and it is called systemic acquired resistance (SAR).
3. Several chemical compounds such as salicylic acid, archidonic acid and 2.6- dichloroisonicotinic acid may induce localized and systemic

resistance in plants at levels not causing tissue necrosis.

4. Such chemicals may be effective in inducing resistance in plants when they are applied through the roots, as a foliar spray or stem injection.

4.1. Characteristic of LAR

- LAR results in near absence of lesions immediately next to the existing lesion.
- Smaller and fewer local lesions developing farther not from the existing local lesions when inoculations made at least 2-3 days after the primary infection.
- LAR limit the number and size of lesions per unit area.
- Eaxample: LAR is induced in a 1to 2 mm zone around local lesions caused by TMV on hypersensitive tobacco varieties and probably in other host combinations.
- It is very important for plants to combat biotrophic pathogens, such as *Peronospora parasitica*, *Pseudomonas syringae*, and Erysiphe spp., by restricting their access to water and nutrients .

4.2. Characteristic of SAR

- SAR acts nonspecifically throughout the plant and reduces the severity of disease caused by all class of pathogens.
- SAR has been studied most in cucurbits, solanaceous plants, legumes, and gramineous plants following infection with appropriate fungi, bacteria and viruses.
- SAR cannot be induced after onset of flowering and fruiting in the host plant.
- SAR is characterized by the coordinate induction in uninfected leaves of inoculated plants of at least nine families of genes known as SAR genes.
- R gene-mediated resistance also activates SA-dependent signaling, leading to an activation of a string of presumed defense effector genes.
- This activation of SA signaling occurs throughout the plant to develop systemic acquired resistance (SAR) against subsequent pathogen infections.
- During SAR, deposition of callose and lignin occurs in the plant cell walls, and plants acquire the ability to mount a rapid HR.

- Products of several SAR genes, for examples, -1-3 glucanases, chitinases, PR-1 proteins, have direct antimicrobial activity or are closely related to classes of antimicrobial proteins.
- SAR does not affect spore germination and appressorium formation. However, penetration is drastically reduced in systemically induced resistant tissue.
- SAR is also characterized by induction of peroxidase and lipoxygenase activities the lead to the production of fatty acid derivatives which exhibit strong antimicrobial activity.
- Salicylic acid and isonicotinic acid are true SAR activators because not only do they induce resistance to the same spectrum of pathogens and induce expression of same genes as do pathogens, but these chemicals have no antimicrobial activities.

Table. Systemic Acquired Resistance (SAR) & Induced Systemic Resistance (ISR)

Features	**ISR**	**SAR**
Definition	Resistance activated in response to artificial application of non pathogenic strains of pathogen, PGPR, and abiotic stresses	Resistance activated in response pathogenic infection.
Pathway	Jasmonic acid dependent pathway	Salicylic acid dependent pathway
Signalling molecule	Jasmonic acid	Salicylic acid
Defense gene involved	CHIB, HEL,PDF1,2	PR-1 and PR-2
Pathogen associated	Operates against biotrophic pathogens	Operate against necrotrophic and facultative parasite

5. Plant defense inducers

- Synthetic compounds which can induce resistance in plants to several viruses , fungi and bacteria are called plant defense inducers.
- They includes salicylic acid and dichloroisonicotinic acid (INA).
- They are applied by injection into the plant, spraying onto leaves or absorption through the petiole or through the roots.
- Such synthetic chemicals reported as effective inducers of systemic acquired resistance against several pathogens like TMV, *Peronospora tabacina* and *Pseudomonas syringae.*
- A great dill of work is going on in these area by public and private sector in developing compounds that would induce SAR to plant disease.

- One such compound known as CGA 245704 that have no antimicrobial activity but mimic the biological induction of SAR in both dicot and monocot crops against many pathogens.

6. Gene editing

- Gene editing is an exciting innovation that has captured the imagination of the research community, which allows scientists to make more targeted improvements within a plant's DNA to produce a disease and pest resistant crop.
- It has the potential to solve real challenges for farmers and the planet, like reducing the need for pesticides and the use of energy, land, and water.
- In agriculture, this process typically looks to improve a beneficial trait within an organism or to remove an undesirable trait .
- For years, "gene editing" was done through selective breeding in plants. But now we can make changes with more precision than ever before.
- Gene editing tools, like CRISPR, are already helping researchers to make improvements within plant DNA .
- These tools enable scientists to deactivate unfavorable traits, such as disease vulnerability and support beneficial traits, such as drought tolerance or improved nutrition.
- These tools have the potential to offer unmatched precision to farmers, allowing them to grow enough food while confidently reducing their use of natural resources.
- By giving plants a better chance at survival—particularly in regions that struggle with hunger and malnutrition—gene editing can give people a better chance at life.

7. Molecular mechanisms underlying activation of plant defense responses

- Molecular mechanisms underlying activation of plant defense responses are quite different between biotrophs and necrotrophs.
- Plant defense against biotrophic pathogens is largely due to gene-to-gene resistance.
- R gene-mediated resistance usually results in hypersensitive response (HR).

- It is very important for plants to combat biotrophic pathogens, such as *Peronospora parasitica, Pseudomonas syringae*, and Erysiphe spp., by restricting their access to water and nutrients .
- R gene-mediated resistance also activates SA-dependent signaling, leading to an activation of a string of presumed defense effector genes.
- This activation of SA signaling occurs throughout the plant to develop systemic acquired resistance (SAR) against subsequent pathogen infections.
- During SAR, deposition of callose and lignin occurs in the plant cell walls, and plants acquire the ability to mount a rapid HR.
- Analysis of Arabidopsis mutants with defects in various defense-related signaling pathways provides support for the idea that SA signaling can result in resistance to biotrophic pathogens.
- For instance, both EDS1 and PAD4 play important roles in SA signaling, and mutations in these two loci weaken resistance to some *Peronospora parasitica* isolates.
- The NPR1 (Nonexpressor of pathogenesis-related genes 1) gene is a master regulator for SA signaling. The npr1 mutant is more susceptible to a variety of pathogens .
- Mutants with defective SA synthesis, including eds5 and sid2 show enhanced susceptibility to *P. syringae.*
- Two plant-specific DNA- binding proteins, SAR Deficient 1 (SARD1) and CBP60g, are key regulators for SA synthesis. Knocking out SARD1 compromises basal resistance and SAR.
- In the sard1-1/ cbp60g-1 double mutant, pathogen-induced SA synthesis are blocked in both local and systemic leaves, resulting in compromised basal resistance and loss of SAR.
- In addition, the expression of CBP60g/SARD1- dependent resistance-related genes are modulated by 25Y.

15

Marker-Assisted Selection

1. **Markers:** Easily identifiable features are called markers or marker features.

2. **Types of marker**

These markers are three types

2.1.Morphological markers: These relate to the size, shape, color and surface area of different parts of the plant.

2.2.Biochemical markers: Such markers refer to changes in protein structure. For example, isozymes and storage proteins.

2.3.Molecular marker or DNA markers: Refers to a unique nucleotide sequence found on a DNA strand.

3.Common features of DNA markers

General characteristics of DNA markers are outlined below.

- Markers are easily recognizable or identifiable.
- Markers serve as red flags or markers for the presence of the gene of interest.
- DNA markers are useful or used in marker-assisted selection (MAS).
- The marker is very close to the gene of interest.
- Markers are gene-associated and are most often inherited along with the gene.
- DNA markers can be used to identify corresponding genes in distant plant species as well as animal and microbial species.

4. Types of DNA markers

There are different types of DNA markers. DNA markers used in plant pathology are listed below.

4.1. Hybridization-based markers

- Random fragment length polymorphism (RFLP)

4.2. PCR-based markers

- Randomly amplified polymorphic DNA (RAPD)
- Microsatellite (SSR)
- Amplified fragement length polymorphism (AFLP)

4.3. Sequencing - based markers

- Single nucleotide polymorphism (SNP)
- Internal transcribed spacer (ITSs)

Table : Comparison of the five most widely used DNA markers in plant pathology

Particulars	**RFLP**	**RAPD**	**AFLP**	**SSR**	**SNP**
DNA required(μg)	10	0.02	0.5-1.0	0.05	0.05
Quantity of DNA	High	High	Moderate	Moderate	High
PCR based	No	Yes	Yes	Yes	Yes
Number of polymorphism loci analysed	1-3	1.5-50	20-100	1-3	1.0
Prior information needed	Yes	No	No	Yes	Yes
Ease of use and development	Not easy	Easy	Easy	Easy	Easy
Reproducibility	High	Unreliable	High	High	High
Cost analysis	High	Low	Moderate	Low	Low
Automation	Low	Moderate	Moderate	High	High
Accuracy	Very high	Very low	Medium	High	Very high
Radioactive detection	Usually	Yes	No	No	Yes

5. Application of molecular markers in genome analysis of plant pathogens

1. Gene mapping and tagging.
2. Identification of pathogenic species or strains of plants.
3. Genetic structure.
4. Polymorphism and genetic diversity.
5. Taxonomy and phylogeny.

6. Marker Assisted Selection (MAS)

Marker-assisted selection (MAS) is an indirect selection process in which traits (eg, productivity, disease resistance, abiotic stress tolerance, and/or quality) are targeted. Selection is not based on the trait itself, but on markers associated with it (based on morphological, biochemical, or DNA/RNA markers). For example, when MAS is used to select individuals with disease, the extent of disease is not quantified, but disease-associated marker alleles are used to determine the presence of disease. The assumption is that the linked alleles are associated with a gene of interest and/or a quantitative trait locus (QTL). MAS may be useful for traits that are difficult to measure, have low heritability, and/or are expressed late in development.

Table : Comparison of MAS and Phenotypic Selection

Sl.No	Particulars	Marker Assisted Selection	Phenotypic Selection
1	Markers used	Molecular markers	Morphological markers
2	Laboratory required	Sophisticated	Simple laboratory
3	Technical skill required	Very high	Medium
4	Accuracy	Very high	Medium to high
5	Time required to release a variety	Very short (3-5 years)	Very long (10-15 years)
6	Cost involved	Very high	Low to medium
7	Environmental effect	No effect	Very high
8	Effect of gene interaction	No effect	Very high
9	Mapping of QTL	Possible	Not Possible

6.1. MAS procedure

Marker-assisted selection consists of five critical steps

6.1.1. Selection of parents

- Parents with contrasting characters or different backgrounds should be selected.
- Parent selection requires examining the germplasm to select parents with different DNA.
- Parents used for MAS must be pure (homozygous).
- In self-pollinating species, the plants are usually homozygous. In cross-pollinated species, inbred lines are used as parents.

6.1.2. Development of breeding populations

- This is his second step in applying marker-assisted selection.
- Cross the selected parent to get F_1 plant.
- F1 plants between two pure-bred or inbred lines are homozygous but heterozygous for all RFLPs from the two parents involved in the F_1.
- F_2 progeny are required to study RFLP segregation patterns.

- In general, 50–100 F_2 plants are sufficient to investigate RFLP marker segregation.

6.1.3. DNA isolation

- The third step is the isolation of DNA from the breeding population.
- Isolate DNA from each plant in the F_2 population.
- Digest the isolated DNA with specific restriction enzymes to obtain DNA fragments.
- Subject the digested DNA to agarose gel electrophoresis to separate the different sized DNA fragments.
- Gels are stained with ethidium bromide, and changes in DNA fragments are visible under UV light.
- Nuclear DNA of higher plants produces millions of fragments in a contiguous range of sizes when digested with specific restriction enzymes.
- Digestion of chloroplast DNA with specific enzymes produces approximately 40 fragments of varying sizes.

6.1.4. Evaluation of RFLP

- RFLP polymorphisms between parents and recombinant involvement in the F_2 population are determined using DNA probes.
- Labeled probes are used to find similar fragments.
- Probes hybridize only to segments that are essentially complementary.
- 32P is commonly used for radiolabeling of DNA probes.
- Non-radioactive probe labeling techniques are now available.
- This is how RFLP is determined.

6.1. 5. Correlations with morphological features

- DNA markers correlate with morphological markers confirming indirect selection by molecular markers.
- Once correlations between molecular and morphological markers are established, MAS can be effectively used to genetically enhance various economic traits.

6.2. Advantages of MAS

- Accuracy.
- Rapid method.
- Non-transgenic product.
- Early detection of traits.
- Screening of difficult traits.
- Gene pyramiding.
- Small sample for testing.
- Permits QTL mapping.
- Highly reproducible.

6.3. Limitation of MAS

- MAS is an expensive method.
- A well-equipped laboratory is required.
- MAS requires well-trained personnel.
- Detection of various bound DNA markers (AFLP, RFLP, RAPD, SSR, SNP, etc.) is a difficult, tedious and time-consuming task.
- MAS may use radioactive isotopes to label DNA, which can lead to serious health hazards.

6.4. Practical Achievements

- MAS was mainly used for developing disease-resistant varieties in various crops (Table 1).
- In rice, MAS has been successfully used to develop cultivars resistant to bacterial blight and blast.
- For bacterial blight resistance, four genes (Xa4, Xa5, Xa13, Xa21) were arranged in a pyramid using STS markers. Pyramidal lines showed higher levels of resistance to bacterial pathogens.
- In Indonesia, two rice varieties are resistant to bacterial blight. Angke and Conde were released by MAS.
- For blast resistance, the three genes (Pi1, Piz 5, and Pita) were pyramidalized in susceptible rice cultivar Co39 using RFLP and PCR-based markers.

- Nematode-resistant lines were developed in soybean *via* SSR markers.
- In vegetable crops, MAS in tomato and potato based on RFLP, RAPD and AFLP markers are mainly used for disease resistance.
- In fruit trees, MAS is mainly used for disease resistance in pomegranate, apple and pear based on RFLP, RAPD, SSR and AFLP markers.

Table : Disease resistant character being used for MAS in different crops

Crop	**Disease Resistance**
Rice	Bacterial blight , Blast , Rice tungro virus
Maize	Northern corn blight
Wheat	Leaf rust, Powdery mildew, Loose smut
Soybean	Mosaic virus, Cyst nematode
Pea	Powdery mildew, Fusarium wilt
Tomato	Bacterial wilt, Black mold, Yellow leaf curl virus
Potato	Late blight,Potato virus X
Barley	Powdery mildew, Stripe rust,
Sunflower	Downy mildew

16

Genetic Engineering for Disease Resistance

Introduction

Genetic engineering is the process of using molecular techniques to add, modify and delete genes of interest to the DNA strands of recipient cells or recipient plants. Genetic engineering is also called genetic technology, transgenic technology, transformation technology and recombinant DNA technology. Genetic engineering consists of tools and techniques used to study, identify, or modify the genes of living organisms. It is also defined as a technique for developing transgenic organisms. The key points of genetic engineering are briefly listed below.

1. Transgene

- A genetically engineered or genetically modified gene is called a transgene.
- Such genes are used by another unrelated plant or organism.
- May come from microorganisms (viruses, bacteria, fungi), unrelated species or animals.
- A transgenic individual therefore contains some DNA from another organism.

2. Transgenic

- A genetically modified organism or individual is called a transgenic.
- The term transgenic was first used by Gordon and Ruddle in his 1981.
- A plant containing a transgene is called a transgenic.
- Transgenic crops contain one or several genes that have been artificially inserted to bypass the sexual process.
- Transgenic individuals contain new genes introduced by genetic engineering.

3. Transgenic technology

- Techniques or processes used to develop transgenic individuals are called transgenic techniques.
- Plant breeders/plant pathologists can combine useful genes from different organisms into one plant.
- Providing a means of identifying and isolating the genes that control specific traits in one type of organism and transferring those genes to another, completely different organism with those traits.

4. Recombinant DNA technology

- Recombinant DNA technology refers to a set of techniques used to isolate DNA from one organism, modify it, and integrate it into the genome of another individual or organism.
- Recombinant DNA is hybrid or chimeric DNA that can combine with the DNA of any organism.
- Same as genetic engineering.

5. Gene cloning

- A genetic engineering technique in which a genetic sequence is propagated in many identical copies.
- Identical gene sequences are separated using restriction endonuclease enzymes.
- This can be obtained by using reverse transcriptase to generate complementary DNA from an mRNA template.
- It is then transformed into a cloning vector like plasmid or bacteriophage.
- Plasmids are used to infect cells (plants or bacteria) and replicate within the cells.
- Gene cloning is used to identify the molecular structure of genes.

6. Gene sequencing

- Gene sequencing is the determination of the order of bases in the DNA molecules that make up a gene.
- DNA is purified and cleaved at specific sites with enzyme restriction endonucleases.
- Therefore, the ends of all strands are identical.

- These strands are then cut at random distances from their ends, strands ending at each existing base.
- Then separate these strands, identify their terminal bases, sort by fragment size, and determine the entire sequence.

6. Gene splicing

- Enzyme-catalyzed joining of DNA fragments is called gene splicing.
- This occurs within the cell nucleus and is catalyzed by splicing enzymes such as ligases.

7. DNA probe

- A small segment of DNA with known sequence, origin and function is called a DNA probe.
- DNA probes can be obtained from DNA templates or generated by gene cloning techniques.
- Sophisticated microprocessor-based devices called 'genetic synthesizers' are available to create DNA probes.
- Useful for determining nucleotide sequences in non-living systems as well as in living systems.

8. Southern blotting

- The method used to detect the presence of specific DNA sequences is called southern blotting.
- This technique was developed by Edwin Southern in 1975.
- Also known as southern blot, southern transfer, southern hybridization, and DNA gel blot analysis.
- This technique is often used to detect specific DNA fragments in complex mixtures.

9. Northern blotting

- Methods used to determine the presence of specific mRNAs from mixtures of RNA.
- This technique was developed by Alwine and his colleagues in 1977 and further developed by Thomas in 1980.
- Also known as northern blot, northern transfer, and RNA gel blot analysis.

10. Western blotting

- A method used to detect the presence of a particular protein in a sample using an antibody specific for that protein.
- This technique was developed by Ipwbin and colleagues in 1979.
- This technology uses antibodies to detect specific proteins.
- Used to detect the presence of specific proteins in tissue samples.

11. Method of gene transfer

There are four ways to introduce foreign substances (DNA) into crops. These are

(1) Plasmid method

(2) Particle impact method

(3) Direct uptake of DNA

(4) Microinjection

These are briefly described below.

1. Plasmid method

- This is an agrobacterium-mediated technique for exogenous gene transfer.
- Also known as biological methods of gene transfer.
- The main features of this method are listed below.
  - Regeneration from cells or protoplasts is required for usage in cell or protoplast culture.
  - Transformation method cheaper than gene gun method.
  - Some control over transgene copy number and integration site.
  - The main drawback of this method is host specificity, somatic mutations and slow regeneration.

2. Particle bombardment method

- In this method, foreign DNA is inserted into plant cells *via* gene gum using DNA beads coated with gold or tungsten.
- Also called particle acceleration microballistic method.

- The main features of this method are listed below.
    - This method is simpler than the plasmid method and is not host-specific.
    - Used in meristems, immature embryos, embryogenic callus, suspensions and hypocotyls.
    - This approach can't be employed since gene guns are so expensive.
    - It is not possible to control the copy number and location of the foreign gene integration.

3. Direct DNA transfer

- This method involves electroporation and is used with protoplasts.
- Regeneration from protoplasts is therefore a fundamental requirement of this method.
- This method is of limited use.
- The main features of this method are:
    - An inexpensive method of exogenous gene transfer.
    - Used in protoplast culture.
    - Host-specific.
    - Slow recovery.

4. Microinjection method

- In this method, plasmid DNA is introduced into host cells through a microscope needle, known as microinjection.
- The main features of this method are listed below.
    - Used in protoplast culture.
    - It has no host specificity.
    - Protoplast regeneration is slow.
    - It is an inexpensive exogenous gene transfer method.

Of these, the first two of this methods, the plasmid method and the gene gun method, are used for the development of transgenic crops. The other two methods are less commonly used.

12. Detection of transgenes by selectable marker technology

- A selectable marker is added to the target gene for easy identification of the gene of interest.
- Antibiotic resistance genes are commonly used as selectable markers to determine if the new gene has been introduced into the host plant.
- The kanamycin resistance gene is used to identify transformed cells.
- A lethal concentration of kanamycin is added to plasmid (bacterial) mixture suspensions or protoplast cultures.
- Non-transformed cells die and only transformed protoplasts survive.
- This helps detect transformed cells.

PCR, ELISA, Southern blot, Northern blot, and Western blot techniques are also used to detect transformed cells. Only transformed cells are regenerated into whole plants to further test the stability of gene expression.

13. Steps in the genetic engineering process (transgene technology)

1. Identification of useful genes

- This work is done in a laboratory.
- The gene of interest can be found in wild species, unrelated plant species, and unrelated organisms, microorganisms (bacteria, viruses or fungi) and animals.

2. Design of inserted gene

- The gene of interest is isolated from the donor and cloned in the laboratory.
- Cloning is usually done using plasmids.

3. Insertion of the gene into the target plant

- A cloned gene, i.e. multiple copies of the gene of interest are introduced into the host or recipient plant.
- Two ways. Agrobacterium-mediated and gene gun or particle bombardment methods are used for gene transfer.
- The plasmid method uses protoplast cultures and the gene gun method uses meristematic tissue or embryogenic callus.
- This happens in the lab.

4. Identification of transgenic cells

- Transformed cells are identified using a selectable marker (kanamycin) and regenerated into whole plants in culture medium.
- Regenerated plants are compared to the parent variety.
- It should look like the parent strain, except for the gene of interest.
- This work takes place in laboratories and greenhouses.

5. Small scale field test

- Performance of transgenic plants is evaluated in small field trials.
- Seeds of transgenic plants such as cotton, soybeans, and rapeseed etc. is tested in laboratory for biosafety i.e allergenicity and toxicity.
- These studies are performed on animals such as rabbits, poultry and goats.

6. Large scale field test

- Regulatory approved transgenic plants are evaluated in a multi-location trail for their performance for the gene of interest.
- Good performing genotypes are released after testing and have stable performance for 3 years.

14. Advantages of transgenic technology

The main advantages of this approach are:

- Increased yield and productivity through disease control.
- Reduced cultivation costs due to reduced use of chemicals.
- Reduce the use of pesticides to reduce pollution.
- Breeding of beneficial insects i.e natural enemies and parasites of pests. In other words, the transgene does not adversely affect the beneficial insects.
- Therefore, genes that confer resistance are environmentally friendly. As a result, there is no risk of harm to human or animal health.

15. Disease control using transgenic plants

- Modern DNA technology allows the production of transgenic plants resistant to certain diseases.

- Use of coding enzymes such as chitinases and glucanases that target specific groups of pathogens such as fungi, viruses and bacteria.
- Use of nucleic acid sequences that lead to gene silencing of pathogens.
- Resistance to negative environmental influences.

16. Transformation techniques for transgenic plants

1. Transgenic plants transformed with specific plant genes for resistance.
2. Transgenic plants transformed with genes coding for antipathogen.
3. Transgenic plants transformed with nucleic acids that lead to resistance and to silencing of pathogen genes.
4. Transgenic plants transformed with combinations of resistance genes.
5. Transgenic plants producing antibodies against the pathogens.

1. Transgenic plants transformed with specific plant genes for resistance

- There are many crops in which plant genes for specific pathogens have been isolated from resistant plants, transferred to susceptible plants and expressed in those plants.
- Necessary support genes are also transferred to the new host and expressed.
- Some previously susceptible plants now behave like tolerant plants.
- Examples of crops transformed with plant resistance genes.
    - Hybrid rice transformed with the rice gene Xa21, which encodes rice resistance to bacterial blight caused by *Xanthomonas oryzae pv. oryzae*.
    - Introduction of the resistance gene DRR206 from peas into rapeseed resulted in transgenic rape resistant to blackleg caused by the fungus *Leptosphaeria maculans*.
    - Reduced seedling mortality from the root pathogen *Rhizoctonia solani* and reduced leaf lesions from *Sclerotinia sclerotiorum.*
    - Similarly, in crooked grass plants transformed with the Arabidopsis gene PR5K, which encodes a protein kinase receptor whose extracellular domain resembles the PR5 family of pathogenesis-related (PR) proteins.

- Transgenic plants show resistance to the fungus *Sclerotinia homeocarpa*, which causes dollar spot disease, with disease symptoms delayed by 29 to 45 days.
- When tobacco and many other plants were transformed with animal anti-apoptotic genes, the plants became resistant to necrotic pathogens, whereas transgenic plants in which this gene was disrupted it did not protect against pathogens.

2. Transgenic plants transformed with genes coding for antipathogen

- Composite genes encoding multiple pathogenesis-related (PR) proteins, including chitinases and some glucanases.
- They are isolated, cloned and expressed in plants to interfere with the development of specific groups of pathogens and confer resistance to affected plants.
- Examples of plants transformed with genes encoding antipathogenic compounds are:
    - Peanut plants transformed with an antifungal gene that reduces the incidence of sclerotinia rot caused by *Sclerotinia minor*.
    - Transgenic rose plants expressing a chitinase transgene from rice showed reduced symptoms caused by the fungus *Diplocarpon rosae*, the cause of black spot in roses.
    - Transgenic broccoli plants expressing the endochitinase gene from the biocontrol fungus *Trichoderma harzianum* had endochitinase activity 14- to 200-fold higher than controls and exhibited significantly milder symptoms than non-transgenic plants.
    - Transgenic cotton and tobacco plants expressing the glucose oxidase gene from the biocontrol fungus *Talaromyces flavus* show significant seedling resistance to Rhizoctonia and partial resistance to Verticillium. However, it showed no resistance to Fusarium.
    - Glucose oxidase unfortunately produces hydrogen peroxide which is toxic to both pathogens and plants.
    - Transgenic *A. thaliana* plants expressing one or both of the genes encoding cysteine protein inhibitors, or, to a lesser extent, cowpea trypsin (serine) protein inhibitors, protect plants from infection by various species of nematodes like *Rotylenchus reniformis*.

- The increased resistance shown in transgenic tobacco plants overexpressing the glutamate decarboxylase gene renders the plants resistant to root-knot nematodes.
- Transgenic tobacco and potato expressing the bacterial gene ubiC, which leads to accumulation of the toxic 4-hydroxybenzoic acid glucoside.
- Oilseed rape (*Brassica napus*) expresses an antimicrobial peptide that makes the plant resistant to blackleg caused by the fungus *Leptosphaeria maculans.*
- A peanut plant transformed with a gene encoding an antifungal enzyme that renders the plant resistant to *Sclerotinia sclerotiorum.*

3. Transgenic plants transformed with nucleic acids that lead to resistance and to silencing of pathogen genes

- Insertion of viral or other nucleic acid segments into the plant genome often silences genes of viruses or subsequent pathogens with homologous sequences, rendering plants resistant.
- There are several well-documented cases of successful transformation of susceptible crops into resistant crops by genetic engineering using parts of the viral genome.
- The first example of tobacco that has been transformed with the coat protein gene of Tobacco mosaic virus and acquired resistance to that virus.
- For example,
- Insertion of untranslatable coat protein
    - Insert the untranslatable Tobacco etch virus (TEV) coat protein coding sequence.
    - Produces transgenic plants that develop symptoms on inoculated leaves.
    - However, the rest of the plant remains asymptomatic.
- **Insertion of double-stranded RNase gene**
    - Insert the yeast-derived double-stranded RNase gene into the genome of the pea plant.
    - It has made transgenic pea plants resistant to several viruses.

- **Transformed with coat protein genome**
  - Pumpkins transformed with coat protein genomes of cucumber mosaic, and watermelon mosaic viruses.
  - Papaya transformed with the papaya ringspot virus envelope protein gene.
  - Soybean transformed with soybean mosaic virus CP nucleic acid.
  - Tobacco containing tobacco leaf spot virus.
- **Viral nucleic acids used to transform plants**
- **For example**
  - Peanut plants were transformed to confer resistance to tomato spot wilt virus by conferring an antisense nucleocapsid gene sequence.
  - Transgenic potato plants integrate the antisense orientation of the P1 gene into the potato genome became highly resistant to potato virus Y.
- **Viral replicase genome**
  - Transformation by introducing the viral replicase gene into the genome.
  - Successfully transformed plants such as wheat, potato, tomato, cucmber with viral replicase gene and made the transgenic plants resistant to multiple viruses.
  - Examples include transgenic wheat infected with wheat streak mosaic virus, potato leaf roll virus in tomato, tomato yellow leaf curl virus and cucumber mosaic virus, potato leaf roll virus in potato and potato virus Y.
- **Motor protein gene**
  - Using motor protein genes from raspberry bush dwarf virus in raspberry, tobacco mosaic virus in tomato, and cymbidium mosaic virus in dendrobium.
  - Genes encoding viral inclusion bodies in plant cells.
  - Genes encoding various nonstructural proteins of the virus.
- **Non-viral genes**
  - Successfully transformed plants such as wheat, potato, peas, tobacco and walnuts with non-viral genes and made the transgenic plants resistant to multiple viruses.

- Non-viral genes that confer resistance to viruses include the Schizosaccharomyces pombe double-stranded RNase (dsRNase) gene.
- Tobacco resistance gene N, mouse protein kinase, systemically acquired tobacco resistance gene 8.2, etc.

- **Defective interfering DNAs or RNAs**
  - Resistance to viruses is mediated by small defective interfering DNA or RNA.
  - Occur naturally in plant cells or produced after inoculation with DNA or RNA viruses or transgenes.
  - These small pieces of DNA and RNA are involved not only in silencing the virus, but also in silencing other genes in infected cells.
  - In general, the transgene should be stable.
- **Inactivation of transgene activity can occur either**
  - Lack of transcription, possibly as a result of promoter region DNA methylation and chromatin condensation.
  - By transcript instability (post-transcriptional silencing) as a result of the initiation of RNA degradation processes affecting the transgenic RNA and its homologous RNA.

4. Transgenic plants transformed with combinations of resistance genes

- Broad and effective resistance in many host/pathogen combinations is provided by combination of host genes for resistance with pathogen-derived defense genes or genes encoding antimicrobial compounds.
- Transgenic rice with host gene and promoter and the first intron of the maize ubiquitin gene confers resistance to rice blast (*Magnaporthe grisea*).
- Combination of tobacco host genes and tobacco vein spot virus coat protein genes that exhibit broad and potent resistance to tobacco potyviruses.
- Combination of the Sw5 tomato gene and the nucleocapsid (N) protein gene of TSWV for resistance to tomato spotted welt virus (TSWV) in transgenic plants.

5. Transgenic plants producing antibodies against the pathogens

- Plants do not have the mechanism to produce antibodies.
- However, DNA technology has made it possible to transform plants with additional genes that enable the production of functional recombinant antibodies.
- Such plant antibodies, so-called plant antibodies, may be complete antibody molecules.
- Fab fragments or single chain Fv (scFv) fragments generated against a specific plant virus and directed against the same virus.
- scFv fragments are expressed in the intracellular space and can more effectively increase plant resistance to specific viruses.
- Several plant viruses have been shown to be suppressed in genetically transformed transgenic plants.
- Whole antibodies or single-chain variable region fragments of antibodies can be generated.
- These viruses include Tobacco mosaic virus, Potato virus x, Potato virus y, and Clover vein virus.
- Much more work needs to be done before this method of controlling crop diseases is truly effective and widespread.

Table : Improved disease resistance in transgenic plants overexpressing defense related R genes

Plant	Gene/QTL	Phenotype
Wheat	Lr21	Leaf rust resistance
	Lr10	Leaf rust resistance
Rice	Xa1	Bacterial blight resistance
	Xa4	Bacterial blight resistance
	Xa21	Bacterial blight resistance
	Pi-b	Blast resistance
	Pi-ta	Blast resistance
	$Pi\text{-}k^h$	Blast resistance
Flax	L^6	*Melampsora lini*
	M	*Melampsora lini*
Tomato	Prf	*Pseudomons syringae* pv. tomato
	L^2	*Fusarium oxysporurm*
	Pto	*Pseudomons syringae* pv. tomato
	Cf-9	*Cladosporium fulvum*
	Cf-2	*Cladosporium fulvum*
Potato	StVe	Verticillium wilt resistance
Soybean	SCN	Soybean cyst nematode

Plant	Gene/QTL	Phenotype
Tobacco	N	Tobacco mosaic virus
Sugarbeet	$HS1^{Pro\text{-}1}$	*Heterodera schachtii*
Maize	Hml	*Cochliobolus carbonum,* race 1
Indian Mustard	Ac2(t)	White rust resistance
Pea	Er	Powdery mildew

GM Technology

- We cannot ignore the presence of new GM crop breeding technology.
- But to deal with it responsibly is essential.
- Everything associated with science is not against nature .
- In some cases human involvement hastens the process of evolution to arrives upon solutions to problem faced by us.
- A balance is required.
- Neither science nor nature can be ignored.
- But we must keep on moving scientifically.

GM Crops

- Genetically modified crops.
- Transfer of genes (transgenesis) or gene elements of known function and their integration into random locations along the chromosome of the recipient plant (host plant).
- The donor a related or non related plant, animal or microorganism.

Global metanalysis of impact of biotech crops during 20 years 1995-2014.

Rigorous 2014 meta analysis of European group of 247 data set confirm average benefit are

- 22% increase in yield.
- 37 % decrease in pesticide use
- 65% increase in net profits of farmers.
- Yield and profit gain higher in developing countries than in developed countries.

Source: ISAAA, 2019

Success of GM Crop of India

History of Hybrids

- 1970: First generation ,*G. hirsutum* , intraspecific commercial cotton hybrid released.
- 1983: First interspecific hybrid (*G. hirsutum x G barbedense*) released, followed by hybrids on all 4 species (G. *arboreum, herbaceum, barbedense, & hirsutum*).

Ist GM hybrids

- 2002: First Bt (*Bacillus thuringiensis*) cotton hybrid released.
- Trait : Resistant to bollworm.

The 2nd GM Crop of India; Bt Brinjal

- Gene involved: Cry1Ac.
- Gene source: *Bacillus thuringiensis.*
- Trait: Resistant to Fruit & shoot borer (FSB) (*Leucinodes orbonalis*).
- Developers: Mahyco, TNAU & USA Dharwad.
- GEAC clearance: 14 Oct. 2009.
- Series of public meeting held in early Ministry of Environment & Forestry.
- Moratorium enforces on general cultivation.

The 3rd GM Crop of India : DMH (Dhara Mustard Hybrid)-11

- Gene involved: Bar gene, Bamase & Barstarled (Called Bamase & Barstar system).
- Two gene from : *Bcillus amyloliquefaciens.*
- One gene from: *Streptomyces hygroscopicus.*
- Better suited to hybridization, resistant to herbicide (Basta).
- Yield increase: 25% without much additional input.
- Developed by Delhi University.
- Approval of GEAC for hybrid seed production.

CRISPR/cas: Future Prospectives

- Promising and safe technology for disease resistance.
- Molecular mechanism of numerous pathosystem is known.
- Possible by modification of single gene.
- Targeted mutagenesis
- Chllenges
- Sustainbility issues under field conditions and elite lines/varieties.
- Durability of disease resistance
- Overcoming issues related to targeted mutagenesis.

Long term success depends on new knowledge for identification of genes as well as of modification.

17

Principles of Plant Disease Management

1. Disease Control vs. Disease Management

- The word control evokes the notion of finality, the final elimination of problems .
- It is impossible to exclude , eliminate or prevent diseases.
- Control is ecologically and practically not possible.
- Although disease control is an established and widely understood concept, there are compelling reasons to replace control with management .
- The term control is fast being replaced by management.
- Management conveys the concept of a continuous process rather than an event accomplished by the application of endogenous factors. .
- Plant pathogens are strategically unique components of ecosystems that must be addressed continuously and strategically.
- Management should be based on the principle of keeping damage or loss below the level of economic damage, or at least minimizing the occurrence above that level.
- This management philosophy must be clearly communicated to producers.
- Nevertheless the word control is not abandoned and still commonly used.

1.1. Difference between disease control & disease management

Sl.No	Disease Management	Disease Control
1	Proactive approach	Reactive approach
2	Preventive in nature	Curative in nature
3	Decision will be taken based on EIL	Decision will not taken based on EIL
4	Selective killing	Non selective killing

5	Foucs on regulation of disease	Focus on eradication of disease
6	Disease addressed conntinuously and strategically	Disease not addressed conntinuously and strategically

2. Essential considerations in disease management

2.1. Economic potential of disease.

2.2. Disease management: an integral component of crop production.

2.3. Disease management and area coverage.

2.4. Disease management and timing of treatment.

2.5. Disease management planning for a crop.

2.1 Economic potential of disease

- Temporal and spatial plant disease situations should not always cause economic damage and therefore may not justify control measures.
- There is a need to clearly assess the potential for plant pathogens or plant diseases to cause economic damage under specific conditions.
- The concept of economic threshold should be clearly known to the producer. In most cases, these parameters are unknown, so growers may be wasting effort and resources trying to control even less destructive diseases.
- Others, by contrast, may allow a devastating disease to develop to intolerable levels before attempting to curb it.
- The goal of disease management is to limit the decline in crop economic returns, and if control measures do not increase profits, no grower may accept the recommendations.

2.2 Disease management: An integral component of crop production

- Most cultural practices influence disease development.
- Modern agriculture manages ecosystems to encourage the growth of single plant species.
- In such cropping and farming systems, developing agro ecosystems are unstable, but survive with the adoption of management practices.
- Decisions like choices of plant type, planting date, planting method, fertilization rates, pesticides, tillage type and frequency, irrigation method and frequency, harvesting method, and plant storage all have an impact on the incidence of plant disease and the resulting damage.

- According to Fry (1987), two important principles emerge from the essential relationship between plant production and disease development.
- First, disease control is most effective when all stages of crop production are considered.
- Second principle is that changes in crop production affect disease management.
- For example, host genotypes substitution or altering cultural practices can alter the activity of some pathogens. Disease management must adapt to changes in these hosts and agricultural climates.

2.3 Disease management and area coverage

- Disease cannot act in isolation.
- For any management plan to be successful, it must be applied broadly and consistently.
- When local growers strictly follow recommended disease control practices for their crops while neighboring growers ignore them. The effect of a given treatment is negated by high disease pressure (inoculation) in adjacent fields.
- To avoid this, large-scale collaborative measures such as spraying dead plants with fungicides are needed.
- Increased chances of success in managing diseases and reduced costs of fighting them.

2.4 Disease management and timing of treatment

- A characteristic of plant diseases, especially those of annual crops, is that the disease is recognized when the damage has already occurred.
- Plants do not warn about their diseases. Also, there is no tissue rejuvenation system.
- When treating plant diseases, most procedures are preventive rather than curative, so the timing of treatment is critical to controlling disease development.

2.5 Disease management planning for a crop

- Management plans for major diseases (such as wheat rust and potato blight) are directed against it without considering other diseases of the crop.

- Plant health management involves meticulous planning in which all diseases of varying importance are considered simultaneously.
- Clearly the second approach, though difficult, is of more practical value to the grower.
- Because growers are interested in increasing the productivity of their crops, they prefer a plan that can protect against any disease threat that may arise in the area.

3 Relationship between features of plant pathogens, disease cycle and disease control

- Knowledge of disease etiology, mode of survival, spread, cycles of inoculum production, host-parasite relationships, and the influence of biotic and abiotic factors will aid in the development and application of effective and economical management measures.
- Properly diagnosing problems results in more effective management and lower costs.
- Knowing the primary inoculum of pathogens helps in choosing appropriate management methods and management pathogens at their most vulnerable stages.
- The wheat loose smut disease cycle indicates that the fungus is internally seed borne. Therefore, the primary inoculum is removed by proper seed treatments that can destroy the fungus that resides inside.

4. Principles of plant disease management

The techniques used in disease management mainly based on two principles,: *Prevention or prophylaxis* and *cure* The first principle prevention includes *disease management tactics applied before infection* i.e., *the plant is protected from disease*. It includes: avoidance, exclusion, eradication, resistant & protection. Second principle curative action: *functions with any measure applied after the plant is infected* i.e., *the plant is treated for the disease*.It includes *therapy*

5. Principles of plant disease control

Prophylaxis	Avoidance	Prevent disease by selecting a time of the year or a site where there is no inoculum or where the environment is not favorable for infection.
	Exclusion	Prevent the introduction of inoculums.
	Eradication	Eliminate, destroy or inactivate the inoculums.
	Protection	Prevent infection by means of a toxicant or some other barrier to infection.
	Resistance	Utilize cultivars that are resistant to or tolerant of infection.
Curative	Therapy	Cure plants that are already infected.

5.1 Avoidance of pathogen :*Avoiding disease by planting at times when or where inoculum is absent or ineffective due to unfavorable environment conditions*. The major aim is to enable the host to avoid contact with the pathogen or to ensure that the susceptible stage of the plant does not coincide with favourable conditions for the pathogen. The main practices under avoidance are

- Choice of geographic area.
- Selection of field.
- Choice of time of sowing.
- Disease escaping varieties.
- Selection of seed and planting stock.
- Modification of cultural practices.

- **Example**
    - The potato cultivation at high altitude is relatively free from viruses, as prevailing environmental conditions do not permit the build-up of vector populations.
    - Similarly, early planting of potato or wheat, in Indo-Gangetic plains, may escape late blight or stem rust damage, respectively.

5.2. Exclusion of inoculum :*Preventing the inoculum from entering or establishing in the field or area where it does not exist.* The main practices under exclusion are

- Seed treatment.
- Inspection and certification.
- Quarantine.
- Eradication of insect vectors.

5.3. Eradication of pathogens: *Reducing, inactivating, eliminating or destroying inoculum at the source, either from a region or from an individual plant in which it is already established.*

- Biological control of plant pathogen.
- Crop rotation.
- Removal or destruction of diseased plant organs.
- Rouging.
- Eradication of alternate and collateral hosts.
- Sanitation.
- Heat and chemical treatment of disease plants.
- Soil treatments.
- Examples:
    - One of the largest eradication campaigns ever was the 1927-35 fight against citrus canker (*Xanthomonas axonopodis*) in the United States. Up to 4 million citrus trees were cut down and burned at a cost of about $2.5 million to eradicate the pathogen.
    - Practices routinely used to destroy inoculum include substitution and/ or host destruction (Barbery destruction in the US).

5.4. **Resistant:** *Utilize cultivars that are resistant to or tolerant of infection.*

- Resistant varieties, If available you can manage disease at zero cost.
- It uses built-in mechanisms to resist various activities of pathogens.
- Infection or resulting damage caused by pathogens can be reversed by genetic manipulation or chemotherapy.
- Host resistance can also be induced using certain biotic and abiotic factors.
- The discovery of Mendelian laws of inheritance and the development of plant breeding techniques have contributed to the development of crop varieties resistant to specific pathogens or pathogen groups.
- Classical breeding methods include selection, mutation, and crossing.
- The use of biotechnological tools such as tissue culture, genetic engineering and protoplast fusion are used to develop resistant cultivars. of various economically important crops/plants.

5.5. Protection measures: *Preventing infection by creating a chemical toxic barrier between the plant and the pathogen* is comes under protection measures

- Chemical treatment.
- Chemical control of insect vectors.
- Modification of environments.

5. 6. Therapy: *Reducing severity of disease in an infected individual.*

- Treatment of infected host plants has been attempted in economically important horticultural crops.
- The principle of fighting plant diseases offers the possibility of curing or rejuvenating diseased host plants using physical and/or chemical means.
- The first five of these principles are primarily prevention (prophylaxis) and form a key component of plant disease management.
- They are applied to plant populations before infection occurs. This remedy is a curative procedure and is used for infected plant populations.

While these principles are valid today, in the context of modern concepts of plant disease management, they have some critical shortcomings like

- The principles of plant disease control are stated in absolute terms like *exclude, prevent* and *eliminate* that imply a goal of *zero disease*. Plant disease control in this sense in not practical, and in most cases is note even possible. Indeed, we need not eliminate a disease; we merely need to reduce progress and keep *disease development below an acceptable level*. Instead of plant disease control, we need to think in terms of *plant disease management*.
- These principles donot take consideration the *dynamics of plant disease*, that is the changes in the incidence and severity of disease in time and space. We need some means of assessing *quantitatively* the effects of various control measures, singly and in combination on the progress of disease.
- Finally, these principles of plant disease control tend to emphasize *tactics* without fitting them into an *adequate overall strategy*.

Does this mean that we should abandon the traditional principles? Of course not; We merely have to fit them into an appropriate overall strategy based on epidemiological principles.

Strategies versus Tactics

The dictionary definitions of the two terms are similar, but generally speaking, *an overall plan for reaching a particular objectives is called strategy*, while the *specific means for implementing a given strategy* are called *tactics*. What is a strategy at one level of focus could be called a tactic at another level of focus

7. Concept of disease control

Under the concept of disease control, these principles fall into five categories :

1.1. Therapeutic management (physical, chemical, etc.)

1.2. Management of the physical environment (cultural control)

1.3. Management of relevant microbiota (biological antagonism)

1.4. Management of host genes (host resistance)

1.5. Handling of chemical substances (chemical control)

18

Principles of Ecological Disease Management

1. Changes in philosophy about plant disease management

- To achieve reasonable and sustainable results crop disease management philosophy should shift focus from
- Management of pathogens (or insect vectors) to managing host plants.
- A single goal of high productivity to multiple goals of high yield, efficiency, quality and safety.

2. Ecological management of plant diseases

- Keys to the sustainable management of plant diseases based on interactions between plants, pathogens, vectors and the environment are;
  - Establish agroecological systems that promote plant growth and development at the population level.
  - Detrimental to the evolution of pathogens and outbreaks of epidemics.
- This management system consists of two main components:
  - Multiple goals (high yield, efficiency, high quality, safety)
  - A dynamic and integrated approach.
- Integrated approaches show promise in overcoming the problems and challenges associated with current crop disease control strategies to optimize economic, environmental and social benefits.

3. Core of ecological plant disease management

- Manipulate the environment of host-pathogen interaction in favor of the host.
- It can be done through a balanced application of RAER strategies.

- RAER stands for acronym Resistance, Avoidance, Exclusion and Remedy.
- RAER strategies should be applied according to the specific conditions of relevant host-pathogen interactions.
- Plant disease control approaches, such as crop rotation, can achieve resistance, prevention, elimination and equating to curative effects.
- Crop rotation may therefore be extended into future agriculture, despite some practical limitations.

3.1. Host resistance

- The most effective and convenient approach to treat crop diseases.
- It can be inductive or constructive, systematic or local, qualitative or quantitative.

3.1.1. Qualitative resistance

- Major gene resistance.
- Very effective.
- Prevent infection.
- Effectiveness may be lost under modern agricultural practices due to increased incidence of plant pathogens.

3.1.2. Quantitative resistance

- Minor gene resistance
- Less effective
- Reducing disease epidemics rather than preventing infection.
- However, they have a longer lifespan due to lower pathogen selection pressure.

3.1.3. Induced drag

- Inductive resistance has an advantage over constructive resistance. This is mainly due to less resource allocation when not needed.

3.1.4. Ten principles of agricultural practices that affect host plant resistance levels

- In addition to the genetics of host resistance, other factors, called the 'Ten Principles of Agricultural Practice', can also affect resistance levels in host plants.

1. Soil
2. Nutrition
3. Water
4. Seeds
5. Population density
6. Crop protection
7. Field management
8. Agricultural machinery technology
9. Light
10. Air

- Altering any of these elements can change the environment in ways that are either beneficial or detrimental to the plant or pathogen.

3.1.5. Host heterogeneity

- One of the most effective ecological approaches to control plant diseases.
- Increased host heterogeneity due to mixed or mixed cultures or cropping.
- Varieties should have different genetic and physiological traits, such as; types of resistance (quantitative vs. qualitative).

- **Benefits**
  - Reduce the spread of disease.
  - Increase nutritional efficiency.
  - Short-term productivity and yield stability.
  - Improves soil fertility.
  - Slows the development of pathogens.
  - Extend the life of resistant varieties.
  - For example:
  - Rice blast control: By growing different rice cultivars, the dependence on the use of fungicides to control rice blast is significantly reduced, while at the same time the quality and quantity of production are greatly increased.

- Potato late blight: It was successfully controlled by using a mixture of different varieties in addition to mixed or capture crop techniques

3.1.6. Other approaches are used to support the ecological management of plant diseases.

3.1.6.1. R gene rotation

3.1.6.2. Gene insertion

3.1.6.3. Gene pyramiding

3.2. Disease avoidance

- Aims to ensure discrepancies between plant critical times and disease onset times.
- Spatial and temporal changes in host plant cultivation patterns.
- This can be done by changing the time of planting, the planting site, or the cultivation system.
- Complex approach that requires full understanding
  - Host susceptibility by different phenological developmental stages.
  - Expected weather conditions.
  - Disease ecology.
  - Distribution of pathogens and pathogen types.

3.2.1. Spatial avoidance

- Efficiency of spatial avoidance, including local use of the R gene and variety mix.
- Primarily determined by pathogen distribution and route of transmission.
- Effective in treating plant diseases caused by soil and waterborne pathogens such as nematodes and bacteria.
- Not suitable for treating airborne diseases that spread over considerable distances in a single epidemic.

3.2.2. Temporary evasion

- These approaches include;

3.2.2.1. Change of planting time

3.2.2.1. Crop rotation.

3.2.2.1. Change of planting time

- Efficacy in combating plant diseases is highly dependent on seasonal climatic conditions.
- This is especially true for polycyclic pathogens where the primary inoculum does not play a significant role in epidemics.
- For rice virus disease, this approach reduces the exposure of plants to the pathogen during the most sensitive period by avoiding the peak phase of vector transmission.

3.2.2.2. Crop rotation

- Expected to be particularly effective in controlling plant diseases caused by soil-borne pathogens.
- Very effective control of potato, banana and tobacco bacterial wilt, sweet potato black rot and root rot.
- Pathogens transmitted by insect vectors such as many viruses.

3.3. Exclusion

- Several methods of eliminating overwintering sites (locus and host) of pathogens and their transmission vectors have significant results in the treatment of plant diseases.
- It also minimizes negative environmental impact by eliminating or reducing inoculum sources.
- It is important to identify an appropriate source of primary vaccination.
- Misidentification of primary inoculum not only reduces management efficiency but also wastes resources.
- Numerous agricultural practices have proven to be highly effective in eliminating or reducing pathogenic inoculum sources.
- This is done by adapting cultivation systems to remove diseased plant tissue, streaky hosts and secondary crops.
- Be at the forefront of these practices.

3.3.1 Crop rotation

- A convenient way to eliminate disease.
- Eliminates pathogens (particularly some soilborne pathogens) and potential hosts.

- Improves soil quality (nutrient balance and physical structure) to support healthier plant populations.

3.3.2. Summer plowing

- Tilling the soil after harvest dramatically reduces the population density of the vector *Nephotettix virescens*.
- Therefore, the viral source of rice tungro disease by reducing the overwintering site of the vector.
- Disease eradication strategies are based on a sound understanding of the various interactions that occur between hosts, pathogens and vectors in ecological and epidemiological settings, taking due account of the economic limits of control.

3.4. Remedy

- Use of pesticides in integrated disease control systems.
- The aim is not to completely eradicate the disease, but to control it to the most appropriate degree given ecological and economic limits.
- Pesticides should be used in conjunction with disease prediction and knowledge of the genetic makeup of pathogen populations.
- Determine the optimum timing and frequency of application and select the type and rate of plant protection agent.
- Successful healing can also be achieved by other approaches, such as natural plant substances with biological regulatory effects.
- For example, protein y3 extracted from edible mushrooms and other microorganisms (Bacillus sp.).
- To ensure the effective use of such biopesticides, a better understanding of their properties and application methods is as important as information on relevant biological properties and pathogen transmission routes.
- For example,
  - Spraying 1-2 doses of viral therapeutics or biological control agents at the seedling stage and growing season of rice not only reduces the population density of pathogenic insects, but also protects the plants from further infection.
  - Combining pesticides with other biotic and abiotic approaches such as biotic agents, soil pH adjustment and UV irradiation have been shown to be highly effective for long-term control of root rot in tomato and lettuce.

19

Digital Crop Protection

1. Introduction

- It is becoming increasingly difficult to find workers to work in agriculture.
- Younger generations do not want to work in plant protection.
- We can see that the average age of farmers is getting older.
- This leaves the fields unprotected from disease and insects and greatly reduces yields.
- Fortunately, this gloomy situation has changed since 2015 thanks to modern technology.
- Digital tools are among the most innovative crop protection tools in modern agriculture.
- A new round of innovation in modern agriculture to help farmers collect data and make crop protection more data-driven.

2. Smart crop protection

- Smart crop protection is a fairly new term.
- Majority of farmers are not familiar with what exactly stands behind it.
- This presentation sheds light onto the concept of smart crop protection and why it is the future of farming.
- Term smart crop protection refers to the usage of technologies like internet of things, sensors, location systems, robots and artificial intelligence on a farm to manage pests.
- The objective is increasing the quality and quantity of crops while minimizing the losses.

3. Technologies used in smart crop protection

Digital penetration in the plant protection is growing at a fast pace . A few popular technologies used in smart crop protection are:

- Web
- Mobile technology
- Drone
- Data analysis
- Artificial intelligence (AI)
- Big data
- Blockchain
- Geographic information systems (GIS)
- Agricultural Internet of Things (AIoT)

With internet and mobile penetration rates of 50% and 79% respectively, it provides farmers with a one-stop, digitally-enabled solution.

4. How has digitisation influenced crop protection

- There are approximately 14 million farmers in over 60 million villages in India.
- It is impossible to reach them from any individual or institution.
- Smartphones can bring technology to large numbers of farmers in remote areas.
- Farmers can find appropriate solutions to their problems by downloading specific apps. You can also get in touch with companies like us by simply sending a picture of the problem to get an exact solution.
- In this way, digitization can go a long way in helping farmers bring technology to their doorstep. Examples like weather forecast, disease prediction, insect outbreak prediction, market price prediction, etc. It is very helpful for farmers.

5. Crop protection toolbox

- There is no uniform crop protection approach.
- Today's farmers have a diverse toolbox at their disposal to minimize pest damage.
- It includes cutting-edge chemical and biological products, advanced data analytics and precision technology.
- While these tools are powerful individually, deployed in a holistic IPM

approach tailored to the farmer's specific challenges, they increase effectiveness while minimizing the environmental impact of agriculture.

- Use tools such as artificial intelligence and object-based detection to more accurately assess soil longevity and detect harmful microorganisms.
- Through data science, we can better model and estimate where harmful pests and environmental pressures are greatest, helping growers protect their crops.
- Data science transforms traditional practices into integrated systems designed for sustainable use.
- Real-time data drives accurate application of resources, while cutting-edge software enables quick and easy analysis of crop management and protection.

6. Digital plant doctors

- Accurate information at the right time is very important in crop protection.
- The ability to quickly identify and control diseases can have a significant impact on farmers' time, resources, and ultimately crop productivity.
- The rise of digitization and data has opened up a wealth of new opportunities for farmers.
- Monitor crop conditions 24/7 using smartphones, remote sensors, satellites, drones and artificial intelligence (AI) tools.

7. Digital survey of the field

Goal

- Get more accurate information about crop density.
- To find out when and where diseases affect crops and what steps farmers can take to control them.
- Use crop protection measures in a timely manner and localize them to areas of the field where they are needed.
- This helps reduce the use of pesticides, saving time and money.

Examples

- If the disease affects only 10 square meters of the entire field, the farmer can ignore the remaining area.

- Using laser scanners and a GPS tracking system it took him two days to survey the surface of the 5-hectare test field, but using drone technology it took him only 20 minutes.
- Sensors placed in the field can also help to make accurate predictions about pest infestation, recognize changes at the right time and enable early intervention.
- Microclimate sensors record soil temperature and moisture and provide information on disease prevalence.

8. Crop scouting: More tech to use less

- During a plant's development, weed overgrowth disease, and insect infestation are frequent occurrences..
- Farmers should pay special attention to crop health.
- Previously, farmers had to scout crops visually and on foot, which took a considerable amount of time.
- Many farmers today want the latest and most accurate digital tools, advanced analytics, and powerful imaging equipment to help them make more informed decisions.

9. Precision sprayers (See-and-Spray)

- Ensuring farmers use only the amount of crop protection product needed to address the problem.
- Reduce the possibility of overspray.
- Combining this technology with other crop protection practices allows you to apply products in small amounts in a more targeted manner, positively impacting your bottom line.
- A sprayer with this feature can take pictures of crops on the ground and calculate the exact location of pests between crops.
- This information is sent to precise spray nozzles that target pests only and do not affect crops.

10. Drone usage in agrochemical spraying

- Drone is the most promising technologies to emerge from the fourth industrial revolution.
- The use of drones for pesticide spraying could have a major impact on Indian farms.

- Efficient and effective control of highly mobile and invasive pests such as Fall armyworm (FAW) and desert locust.
- Prevent endemic species while maintaining high agricultural productivity.
- Need government support.

10. Smartphone or Tablet; Digital plant doctors

- Powerful digital tools to provide correct information to farmers, especially smallholder farmers in India.
- Rapid and seamless sharing of knowledge and best practices.
- Farmers can collect pest and disease data, get local crop protection advice, and chat with knowledgeable experts.
- The potential to provide smallholder farmers with the same level of data and insight currently available to farmers in developed countries.

11. Artificial intelligence

- Known as machine learning.
- AI tools analyze staggering amounts of data at high speed and feed back in the form of useful insights that help farmers make critical and timely decisions in the field.
- Detect and diagnose crop diseases and pests in real time in the field.
- The ability to quickly identify and control diseases can have a significant impact on farmers' time, resources and ultimately crop productivity.
- For example, satellite and drone imagery and camera sensors can identify small patches of disease-infested fields.
- Farmers act on this information and treat this small area with targeted applications.
- In the past, farmers may not have recognized a crop disease until a very conspicuous area of the field had become infected, necessitating spraying the entire field instead of just treating a small portion.

12. Professional pest management

- Professional crop protection provides farmers with digital tools that help them optimally monitor their fields before specific problems cause damage.
- These digital tools help provide the farmer with due CARE.

- It shifts the mindset towards prevention rather than cure.
- It give farmers the confidence to stay ahead of any challenge.
- This has proven very beneficial to farmers and advisors in the last months of the pandemic.
- These preventative measures and innovative digital tools enable farmers to do the important work of keeping public spaces and crops free of pests, even during closures.
- Going forward, digital tools and innovative solutions will continue to be the driving force in keeping the environment and crops pest-free in a sustainable way.

13. Mobile plant clinic (MPC)

- Now is the time to pay attention to Mobile Plant Clinic (MPC in India).
- This mobile application platform allows farmers to upload pictures of diseased crops.
- A team of crop protectionists provide expert support in diagnosing and managing infected plants.
- Communication between teams and farmers ultimately benefits both parties.
- Farmers are informed about the etiology and management of plant diseases.
- Teams get first-hand information about the leading diseases in the field and where they need to focus their research appropriately.
- The team will also work with agricultural advisors to help disseminate information to farmers and reach out to farmers in very remote areas.
- The team will meet other researchers from around the world, discuss with the team, exchange ideas, make new connections, potentially collaborate and ultimately use their experience to increase farmer efficiency.

14. Coping with the new normal

- Do not rely on cheap mass production or increased use of primary materials.
- Focus on forward-looking crop protection models that must meet a wide range of requirements.

- Field sanitation services, defined yields per hectare at defined quality levels (eg mycotoxin content and protein content) etc. should be given appropriate strategic considerations.
- Pesticide suppliers and researchers should focus on reducing operating costs and reviewing R&D facilities and portfolios to reduce R&D spending.
- Few companies are making significant efforts to redefine their business model.

15. Hyperspectral imaging technology in crop protection

- Hyperspectral Imaging (HSI) is a technology developed by NASA in the United States 30 years ago and now commercially available.
- A drone-mounted camera that helps characterize the chemical and biological properties of plants and soils by analyzing their reflectance properties over a range of narrow spectral bands.
- This technology inherently arguments human vision, diagnosing and correcting factors limiting plant growth in ecosystems early and in real time.
- It is a relatively new technology that is non-destructive, environmentally friendly, highly accurate, and delivers consistent and rapid results.

Agricultural application

- Crop development and health monitoring.
- Early detection of pests helps prevent crop loss.
- Used to control crop pests that damage target crops on farms.
- This can reduce yield loss by up to 20-40% depending on plant type and growth stage.
- Enabling farmers to deploy sensors in their fields to recognize the presence of pests and weeds on their farms and take preventative measures to protect crops and avoid economic loss. I can.
- The environment is also protected, as the use of pesticides and herbicides can be restricted to areas where treatment is required.
- Significantly improved efficiency and accuracy in crop pest detection compared to traditional methods.

15. First Indian hyperspectral imaging satellite (HySIS)

- The first indian hyperspectral imaging satellite (HySIS) was launched from Sriharikota by the Indian Space Research Organization (ISRO) on November 29, 2018.
- HySIS is used in applications for forestry, geology, assessing coastal zones, and environmental research.
- High cost and complexity.

16. Benefits of digitization to farmers

- Weather forecast.
- Predict disease in advance.
- Predicting pest infestations and losses.
- Estimation of market price, etc.
- Overall, digitization could help farmers bring technology to their doorstep.

20

Biological Agriculture: Prioritizing Nature

India's agricultural accomplishment is a global success story

Parameters	Year	
	1947	2022-23
Population	330 million	1417 million
Food grain production	50 Mt	328 Mt
Per capita grain production	151 kg	231 kg
Contrary to Malthus' prediction, which • India's population increased by a factor of 4.25. • Its food production increased by a factor of 6.55.		

Post Green revolution; Some of the most pertinent questions that humanity faces

- Can we sustain our food production ecosystem, while feeding 9 billon people?
- Can we improve farm economics without reversal of soil biodiversity loss and carbon content?
- Can agriculture play an important role in reducing carbon footprints and mitigating the current climate crisis?

Answers to abovementioned questions do not lie in the currently dominating chemical intensive farming practices, which rely too heavily on

- Fossil-fuel –based fertilizers.
- Chemicals for crop protection.
- Mono-cropping can sustain the demand.
- Nor in natural or organic farming which often seen as a counter strategy as it has its own limitations.

Calls for reducing chemical load

- These concerns have been reflected in high profile initiatives such as the *European Commission's (EC's) Farm to Fork Strategy*, Sustainable Use Directive (2009/128/EC) and European Green Deal.
- The EU is preparing to remove 505 pesticides from the market by 2030 and increase organic farming from 8 to 25%.
- These initiatives echo public concerns for greener and safer food systems, and the World Health Organization's commitment to *"minimising the adverse effects of chemicals on human health and the environment by replacing hazardous chemicals with safer alternatives, including non-chemical ones..."*

Agriculture revolution 3.0

- Focus on developing and implementing advanced bio-agricultural practices.
- These include precision farming, organic farming and genetically modified organisms (GMOs) for increased productivity, sustainability and resource efficiency.
- India can revolutionize the bio agricultural sector in the country by harnessing the power of digital and new media technologies.
- Farmers can optimize resource use, minimize environmental impact and increase crop yields.
- These innovations will help establish India as a global leader in sustainable agriculture.
    - Share your knowledge and expertise with other countries.
    - Promotion of international cooperation.
    - Contribute to global efforts to combat climate change and ensure food security.

A solution in biological agriculture

- Biological agriculture (BioAg) or biocontrol, including biopesticides, biostimulants and biofertilizers, is widely touted as a safe alternative to chemicals in agriculture.
- According to market analysts, the BioAg market is estimated at US$12.6 billion in 2022 and is projected to almost double to US$24.6 billion in 2027 (Markets and Markets, 2022).

- This rapid growth rate reflects the widespread and growing demand for biological solutions as the world pushes ever more environmentally friendly innovations.
- BioAg can be used as part of an organic approach to agriculture. This is important as organic sales continue to grow, reflecting consumer demand for chemical-free products.According to available statistics, in 2021 India ranked fifth in terms of the world's organic agricultural land and first in terms of total number of producers (FIBL & IFOAM Year Book, 2020).
- To maintain its strong position as the world's second largest fruit and vegetable producer, India needs to introduce more non-chemical solutions to control crop pests and diseases.
- The need for more farmers to use his BioAg was recognized in 2022 when Indian Prime Minister Narendra Modi declared his support for organic farming to protect farmers from the impacts of climate change.
- He openly called on Indian farmers to reduce their use of chemical fertilizers and pesticides and switch to organic and natural farming instead.
- Prime Minister Narendra Modi has personally identified over 100 of his BioAg products that can be used to support more sustainable approaches.

Biological agriculture:A sustainable path forward

- Biological agriculture is intermediate between chemical farming and organic farming.
- This is a well-thought-out system approach, not a compromise.
- Opportunities exist for the combined use of biologics and chemicals in favor of reducing reliance on chemicals and soluble fertilizers throughout the food ecosystem.
- Requires more consideration than chemical farming, but provides access to the full range of registered microbial substances.
- Farmers can now very easily understand the value that biology brings to the farm.
- Biological agriculture is therefore an integrated farming system.
- Combine the best of historic regeneration practices refined over centuries with the power of the latest scientific discoveries in the field of biologicals.

- Promotes natural biological processes to dramatically improve crop yields.
- Reduce farm costs through carbon sequestration, reduce carbon emissions and mitigate the climate crisis.

Biological agriculture: prioritizing nature

- Biological Agriculture is in harmony with nature.
- We are witnessing a biodiversity apocalypse with 1 million species critically endangered due to the climate crisis and habitat loss.
- Existing soil biodiversity is also deteriorating at an alarming rate, with an estimated 36 billion tons of soil lost each year (Rodale Report on Carbon Sequestration).
- Not all is lost, but there is great hope for the potential of regenerative agricultural practices if done well.
    - Activate topsoil.
    - Improving soil microbial diversity.
    - Buy CO_2 to support climate protection efforts.
    - Increases plant resistance to stress.
    - Improves crop yields over time, resulting in nutrient-rich crops to combat malnutrition.
- Bio agriculture strives to protect the soil through
    - Improving soil microbial diversity.
    - Using nature to prevent crop pests.
    - An improved root system improves nutrient uptake.
    - Building resilience to abiotic stress.
- It is therefore a natural practice for a regenerative farming systems approach.

Dynamics of bio agriculture

- The emergence of regenerative agriculture has heightened the curiosity of farmers and consumers around the world.
- This will not only restore lost soil health, but also reduce emissions of greenhouse gases such as nitrous oxide and methane, while sequestering

carbon dioxide from the atmosphere into the soil. It also provides an opportunity to address the challenge of climate change.

- Agricultural by-products account for approximately 11% of total greenhouse gas emissions.
- Adding cover crops, reducing tillage and taking other measures can help improve soils and improve yields.
- These practices can also generate carbon credits issued by registrars by increasing soil carbon stocks and reducing greenhouse gas emissions, increasingly in demand by large companies.
- Successful provision of carbon credits will depend on historical data to accurately calibrate and validate models for new practices.

The business case for BioAg

- India is shifting its focus to ensuring food and nutrition security through natural and organic farming.
- Fortunately, there are already hundreds of companies operating in his BioAg division in India.
- This should be reflected in the increased production and manufacturing of bio-Ag, which will slowly but surely replace the polluting giants of the past.
- BioAg emerging trends in India and the rest of the world offer a wealth of welcome opportunities for companies involved in this sector.
- However, many challenges need to be addressed if this 'True Green Revolution' is to bring long-term sustainability to agriculture.
- The top three challenges identified by experts over the last 20-30 years are innovation, design and regulation.
- Until recently, we've been making slow progress on all three of his challenges.
- But it's exciting to see a new focus emerge over the last five years or so.
- Perhaps it was a matter of waiting for the right time.

Resolving long-standing challenges

- Cooperation with industry is required to realize and commercialize many of the innovations from science and its spin-off companies.

- Some of the most brilliant technologies of this century were invented by academics and then developed and/or commercialized in collaboration with large commercial enterprises.
- This is now much more widely recognized.
- Organizations such as the World Bioprotection Forum provide platforms that accelerate innovation by connecting industry and academia.
- Formulation has been an issue with BioAg since biopesticides were commercially introduced in the 1980's.
- Biological products are often more 'fragile' than traditional chemicals.
- They must be formulated to ensure survival and integrity during storage, mixing, application, and in the field.
- Modern technology offers many solutions to this, and this is another example of how industry-academia collaboration can help.
- Finally, problems persisted regarding regulatory approval of new natural and safer microbial alternatives.
- Current regulations in most countries, including the European Union (EU) are still too expensive, too slow, and still not suitable for the biological entities under investigation.
- However, it is encouraging that recent changes in countries like brazil are having a dramatic impact on the use of BioAg. This shows how smarter regulation can promote organic and natural farming.
- We are optimistic that a more enlightened approach will be adopted by this jurisdiction, paving the way for broader change in the near future.

The time is now!

- BioAg is the future.,
- The time for Bio Agriculture the 'True Green Revolution', has finally arrived.
- Backed by consumer demand, environmental groups, regulators and governments, there is a unanimous call to reduce chemical use in agriculture and use more sustainable alternatives such as BioAg.
- While it may seem idealistic to think of a future where agriculture is completely chemical-free, it is a dream worth pursuing, and now finally, it seems closer than ever.

How Atmanirbhar krishi helps

- Farmers' understanding of biologicals has grown rapidly over the past two decades.
- We know that most of the beneficial microorganisms in healthy soil have a symbiotic relationship with plants.
- They plays an important role in nutrient solubility and absorption and protects plants.
- Biologicals farmers use carbon from compost, cover crops, livestock manure and crop residues to support soil microbial life.
- They select crop rotation, increase biodiversity, target crops that fix atmospheric nitrogen, and provide a less costly alternative to the most carbon-intensive inputs of chemical farming.
- They use pesticides responsibly and only when necessary.
- Improved trace element availability and soil longevity have been found to significantly reduce or eliminate the need for pesticides and fungicides, and to recombine carbon from crop residues and cover crops into the soil.

Government initiatives & policies

- Through initiatives such as PM-PRANAM and through ATMA that promote alternative agriculture and reduced fertilizer use.
- Government of India continues to encourage farmers to adopt sustainable practices.
- Government of India has also initiated a number of initiatives such as Paramparagat Krishi Vikas Yojana (PKVY) to promote nature-friendly agriculture.
- To discuss new innovations for sustainable agriculture, the ministry of chemicals and fertilizers host a workshop on strengthening the organic agriculture for sustainable food systems and atmanivar bharat on 6 March 2023 in niti bhawan, New Delhi.
- Science, industry, manufacturers and associations discussed various subjects. The national mission for sustainable agriculture (NMSA) is designed to improve agricultural productivity, especially in rainfall areas, with an emphasis on integrated agriculture, water-use efficiency, soil health management and synergistic resource conservation.

- The Indian government recognizes the importance of promoting sustainable agriculture, but still emphasizes environmentally responsible agriculture.

Gains made by digital India mission

- The government of india is one of the pioneers in mainstreaming the use of digital and new media technologies.
- This will enhance the capacity of central and state government agencies through the digital india mission.
- The government of india has developed guidelines such as the india enterprise architecture (IndEA) to ensure seamless data exchange and interoperability between different digital platforms.
- India digital ecosystem for agriculture (IDEA) focuses on creating an enabling environment for the development and deployment of digital solutions for the agricultural sector.

Precision agriculture & decision support systems

- Precision farming uses advanced technologies such as IoT, AI and big data to collect and analyze farm data for better decision making.
- Sensors, drones, and satellite imagery allow farmers to monitor crop health, soil quality, and other environmental factors in real time, so they can make informed decisions about irrigation, fertilization, and pest control.
- This data-driven approach reduces resource waste, increases crop yields and minimizes environmental impact.
- On the supply side, these technologies can help governments develop evidence-based policies and programs that can provide timely support for long-term sustainability and farmer action.

Blockchain based systems and traceability solutions

- Blockchain technology can be used very effectively to build a transparent and secure supply chain system, allowing full traceability of agricultural products.
- By implementing blockchain, stakeholders can ensure the authenticity of bio agriculture produce, promote fair trade practices and enable consumers to make informed decisions.

- Additionally, these systems will ensure more resilient and transparent warehousing and logistics solutions for manufacturers, buyers and even financial institutions.
- In his World Bank funded SMART project in Maharashtra and Kenya's Blockchain for agricultural supply chain project, there are very successful use cases using a blockchain-based warehouse receipt system.

Robotics and Automation

- Robotics and automation technologies can improve the efficiency of the bio farming sector.
- Autonomous tractors, drones and harvesting robots can optimize field operations, reduce the need for manual labor and minimize crop losses.
- In addition, these technologies help farmers work in difficult weather conditions, increasing overall productivity.
- The world bank's innovative agricultural solutions project in Armenia has supported the adoption of robotics and automation technologies in the country's agricultural sector.
- Similarly, FAO's agricultural mechanization strategy aims to promote the use of robotics and automation to improve agricultural productivity around the world.
- The role of new media in disseminating knowledge and fostering collaboration cannot be overemphasized.
- India can share the latest developments in organic farming and agritech through digital platforms, webinars and social media channels, building a strong ecosystem that connects farmers, researchers and entrepreneurs.

Meeting sustainable developmentgoals (SDGs)

- By adopting more sustainable agricultural practices, India can contribute significantly to global objectives, including
  - SDG 2 (Zero hunger)
  - SDG 12 (Responsible consumption and production)
  - SDG 13 (Climate action)
  - SDG 15 (Life on land)
- In this way, India can act as a role model for other countries, demonstrating the transformative impact of sustainable agriculture and

the benefits of a proactive and collaborative approach to addressing the pressing challenges of our time.

- It is imperative that governments, the private sector and all stakeholders work together to create an environment that fosters the development and adoption of cutting-edge agricultural technologies and practices.

Challenges & future forward

Challenges

- Low effectiveness claims.
- Prevalence of inferior products in the market.
- Reduced budget for product development and innovation.
- How to improve the effectiveness of products and agricultural solutions.

Future forward

- Coordinated efforts at government, industry and academic levels are needed to drive innovation, regulation and farmer awareness

Index